How to Teach: A Handbook for Clinicians

SUCCESS IN MEDICINE SERIES

How to Teach: A Handbook for Clinicians

WRITTEN AND EDITED BY

Shirley Dobson MA Dip Ed

WRITTEN BY

Dr Lesley Bromley

Director of Postgraduate Medical Education, University College London Hospitals NHS Trust

Dr Michael Dobson

Hon. Senior Clinical Lecturer, Nuffield Department of Anaesthetics, University of Oxford

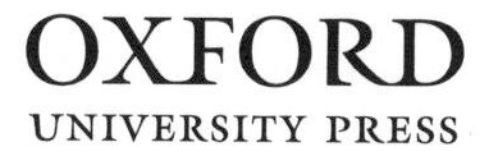
OXFORD
UNIVERSITY PRESS

OXFORD
UNIVERSITY PRESS

Great Clarendon Street, Oxford OX2 6DP

Oxford University Press is a department of the University of Oxford.
It furthers the University's objective of excellence in research, scholarship,
and education by publishing worldwide in

Oxford New York

Auckland Cape Town Dar es Salaam Hong Kong Karachi
Kuala Lumpur Madrid Melbourne Mexico City Nairobi
New Delhi Shanghai Taipei Toronto

With offices in

Argentina Austria Brazil Chile Czech Republic France Greece
Guatemala Hungary Italy Japan Poland Portugal Singapore
South Korea Switzerland Thailand Turkey Ukraine Vietnam

Oxford is a registered trade mark of Oxford University Press
in the UK and in certain other countries

Published in the United States
by Oxford University Press Inc., New York

British Library Cataloguing in Publication Data
Data available

Library of Congress Cataloging in Publication Data
Data available

Typeset in Charter by Glyph International Bangalore, India
Printed in Great Britain
on acid-free paper by
CPI Anthony Rowe, Chippenham, Wiltshire

ISBN 978–0–19–959206–7

10 9 8 7 6 5 4 3 2 1

This book is dedicated to

our friend and supporter Dr Angela Enright.

Acknowledgements

We would like to thank the following for their contributions on simulators:

Dr Mridula Rai
Consultant Anaesthetist, Nuffield Department of Anaesthetics, Oxford

Dr Sarah Chieveley-Williams
Consultant Anaesthetist, Department of Anaesthesia, University College Hospitals NHS Foundation Trust, London

Dr A Hunningher
Specialist Registrar, Department of Anaesthesia, University College Hospitals NHS Foundation Trust, London

We want to thank the following for their scrutiny, ideas, and improvements:

Chapters 3 and 5
Dr Magdalena Mierzewska-Schmidt
Specialist in Anaesthesiology and Intensive Therapy, Warsaw, Poland

Chapters 2 and 12
Dr Gordana Jovanovic
Specialist in Anaesthesia and Intensive Care Medicine, Clinical Centre of Vojvodina, Novi Sad, and Assistant, Faculty of Medicine, University of Novi Sad, Serbia

Chapters 4 and 5
Dr Vojislava Neskovic
Consultant Anaesthetist, Military Medical Academy, Belgrade, Serbia

We would also like to thank Mrs Clare Whyes for advice on use of video in evaluation in Chapter 12.

Contents

Introduction 1: Start here if you want to improve your teaching

Teaching is the best job in the world. Teaching well and inspiring others to teach well is most satisfying. This book is written for you, the busy clinician, so that you can improve your teaching and inspire others.

Good teaching leads to good clinical practice. You learn well from a great teacher because you remember what they taught you. Good teaching in the medical world leads ultimately to better patient care. So a book that helps you to improve your teaching and pass on those skills will be of benefit to patients everywhere. This is a big vision but it is one you can realize.

This book takes you through the stages needed to make you a more effective teacher. It gives you ideas and methods to enable you to keep on improving, even though your main work is clinical. Not everyone is born a gifted teacher, but teaching is a skill like any other that you can learn. As your teaching improves so will your enjoyment of it.

Change is an active process. You are used to updating knowledge and skills in clinical practice. When a new idea comes along, you try it out, discuss the results with others, draw conclusions, and then make plans for the future. So it should be with your teaching: you have some fresh ideas, try them out, get some feedback and discuss them, and then implement this improvement.

Sharing knowledge

No single person has a monopoly of ideas. Ideas and wisdom should be shared. You will find many of the ideas in these pages in other heftier tomes and perhaps little that is original. However, if you follow through step by step you will acquire a fresh way of approaching and delivering your teaching. Many of the educational principles and practices in this book are used in the training of teachers in the UK, and they are fully applicable in all areas of medical teacher training.

Who is this book for?

It is for anyone who passes on their knowledge in the medical world—all clinicians. This book is *not* for you if you are an educational researcher looking for educational theory. It is for those whose primary work is medical, but who have to teach others in the course of their work.

We have used this material widely in the UK, Africa, and South America. Most recently, it has been the basis for an educational programme for a series of courses for young doctors in Central Europe. These doctors have been able to demonstrate to their colleagues through their transformed teaching how much can be learned. Some of them have run their own education training courses.

Worldview, teaching, and culture

Much current literature on adult learning takes into consideration the worldview of the teachers and the learners. Teaching is neither value free nor neutral. We cannot help reflecting our controlling beliefs. We consider fundamental to teaching good relationships with those you teach, knowing when to praise and encourage, and when to challenge.

The content of this book is not culture specific. The practical, educational training methods have been proved effective throughout the world. They aim to give the trainee the appropriate skills to continue to develop their teaching in their own context and culture.

Be creative

Try out ideas yourself and discover new ways of doing things. Good teachers are creative teachers. Talk about your ideas and how you teach with others. The best ideas often grow out of the worst teaching experiences, when you are forced to reflect on what went wrong and come up with something better. Don't allow past failures to depress you. Use them to think about how to do things differently.

A caution

You will find much of this material very basic and obvious. Just because something is simple does not mean it does not work. Beware! There can be a huge gulf between simple ideas and then putting them into practice effectively. We have tried to use straightforward English and avoid jargon. Everything is underpinned by educational theory and some of it is explained in Part 4, but any more than that is the stuff of PhDs, not the purpose of this book.

How to use this book

There are five parts:

Part 1 looks at why we need good teachers.

Part 2 takes you through all stages of preparation and planning for the different ways in which you may present your material.

Part 3 is written to improve your actual teaching skills. We include a chapter on how to teach a clinical skill.

Part 4 gives more detail on the way you can evaluate your teaching and the learning of others. It gives some explanation of how adults learn.

Part 5 is very short but gives you an opportunity to think about your values and your wider vision.

At the end of each chapter, just before the *Notes for Trainers*, we have listed a series of questions for you to think about, because we consider self-evaluation of teaching to be an important aspect of learning to improve. Each chapter ends with *Notes for Trainers*. These are written for those who want to train others using the main content of each chapter.

Some definitions

We realize that you will be teaching a range of people from medical and nursing students, specialist trainees, to senior colleagues. For consistency, in the main content we refer to these learners, or the audience, as the student.

You are reading this book because you want to improve your teaching. Once you begin to notice improvements, we hope you will want to pass this on. That is the point at which you will turn to the *Notes for Trainers* and find all you need on how to run a practical educational course. You can find outlines of sample course programmes and hints on training across languages in the appendices.

As you try out new ideas we hope you and your students enjoy your teaching.

Introduction 2: Read this if you want to run a training course on clinical teaching

This book is written for two audiences. This introduction is for those of you who help clinicians to improve their teaching. Perhaps you want to run a series for your department, you may have done a further education degree and now want to pass on what you have learned to others. You may be running official courses backed by national societies. You will find everything you need to put on and run such a course.

Every chapter is followed by a section entitled *Notes for Trainers*. These notes assume that you have read the chapter and want to use the content. You will find suggested aims, an outline of what to include, and instructions for practical tasks to develop the new skills. Some tasks have specific content, others can be used by any specialty. In the *Notes for Trainers* the learner or course participant is always referred to as a trainee. The trainee may be of any age or at any stage of professional development.

There are sample course programmes in Appendix 2 and they draw on a selection of the core material from different chapters. Whenever you plan a course, it is just like starting to plan an individual teaching session. You must start with your aims and outcomes for the trainees. There are full details on planning and organizing training courses in the *Notes for Trainers* in Chapter 14 How to evaluate a course.

Training at departmental meetings

If you want to offer an education slot once a month in your departmental meeting, plan this carefully. We suggest you begin with the most straightforward, interactive session which leads to the most pronounced changes; this is Chapter 7 Getting your message across. You can follow this with steps for presenting (Chapter 2), some refinements (Chapter 3), improving slides, alternatives to slides (Chapter 6), and becoming a more interactive teacher (Chapter 5).

Having an agreed text

If you are running a course on 'How to Teach' it is very important that every trainee has the same agreed text. This way you are using material appropriate to their specialist area. We recommend the Oxford Handbook series. There are 35 titles and we have indicated in the trainer's notes, when you will find this helpful.

A pattern for an education workshop

Training involves three distinct stages.

- Stage 1

  Short input from the trainer, based on content of the relevant chapter, of up to 20 minutes.

  You must decide whether you will do the teaching interactively, with slides, or without.

  This should take about one-third of the total time.
- Stage 2

  A task or workshop in which the trainees apply or put into practice what they have just heard. You can read in detail how to run these. Below we have outlined some of the things you need to think about when organizing a task or workshop.

  This should take about half the total time.
- Stage 3

  Time to reflect. This takes 5–15 minutes, depending on the level of discussion.

  This is when you give your trainees an opportunity to discuss together what has been different and important for them and time to write down what they personally have learned. It is also the moment when they set themselves a target for their next actual teaching when they will put into practice for real what they have learned.

We follow these stages for every topic on every course. A course based on this book will be practical, as you keep repeating the stages.

Hints on setting tasks

Always plan your task and be flexible with timing until you can predict how long you need. Provide written instructions on paper or on a slide giving the aim, any reference to a handbook, how long trainees will have and exactly what you want them to do. Write down the instructions you will give to explain the task. This sounds overly prescriptive, but it is easy to assume this is straightforward. You especially need to do this if you are working in a second language.

Consider an appropriate size of group for the task you are setting and how you will divide the class.

Follow certain steps.

- Always explain the task and what you want them to have done by the end.
- Give them time to read instructions.
- Ask if there is anything that is not clear.

- Now, and only now, divide them into groups. If you divide people first into groups, they will start to move and will not listen to what you are saying. Tell them where to move to.

The value of practical training

Here is a puzzling question from an education training day that you may share with your trainees: What is the longest distance in the world? After a short pause you give the answer: The distance between your teaching aims and the thoughts of your students. By engaging your trainees through interactive teaching, practical workshops, and reflection, they will make such progress that the distance will be reduced to nothing.

Part 1

The need for good teaching

CHAPTER 1
Why good teachers are necessary

Learning goes on all around us, all the time. We can learn from every patient we see, every procedure we do, every colleague we work with. Our role as a clinical teacher is to make the most of these daily experiences and learn the best ways of passing our knowledge on. Traditionally, teachers were seen as figures of authority and their students sat passively in a class, taking in facts. The assumption made was that once the teacher had spoken, the student would remember everything. This may have served us well for many years but today such methods of teaching and learning are no longer adequate. We face demands from patients, who look to the internet for information and expect high-quality care *and* there is a radical shortening of the hours worked by doctors, which reduces the time for training on the job. We still need good teachers.

'I am a doctor, therefore I can teach'

This statement was put up at a meeting of medical educators in London recently. Unsurprisingly, with such an audience many understood the irony of this statement and disagreed. In a wider group of doctors, there would probably be many who would agree with that statement and assume that teaching came naturally! After all, we have been in full-time education for most of our lives. Since we have seen a lot of teaching, we must be able to do it. This is rather like a Manchester United fan who has never missed a match expecting to be able to play premier league football!

What is a good teacher?

It is sometimes said that great teachers are born. This is wrong; we can all become good teachers. Think of a teacher who was influential in your life and in the career choices you made. Such individuals stand out in our memory.

What are the characteristics that made these people good teachers? Perhaps they were:

knowledgeable
inspiring
funny
interesting
confident
demanding
aware of you.

You may have other characteristics that you can add. All these qualities can be learnt; you can learn how to appear confident; you can learn to be inspiring. You can learn the skills of teaching just as you learn skills in your clinical practice. And you can learn how to improve. You should approach teaching as you approach your clinical work and update your teaching for the 21st century.

Why is good teaching necessary?

Good teaching requires good teachers, the sort of people you have been thinking about. A good teacher is interested not just in good teaching but in the people who are learning. You remember good teachers because of the relationship they built with you as much as for the content. They enthused and motivated you so that you wanted to learn and you remembered what they taught. As changes come thick and fast, those you teach need to be self-motivated to continue to learn and to develop good patterns of learning. These lifelong skills start with good teachers. Good teaching is necessary because you have important information to get across to others who will be working with patients.

Time to stop and think

- Will I be remembered as a good teacher?
- Do I offer a good role model for future teachers?
- Do I motivate and enthuse?
- Do I try to understand my students?
- Do I encourage patterns for lifelong learning?

Notes for Trainers

Why good teachers are necessary

This first talk sets the scene and tone for your education course. It is short, interactive and has very few slides. It contrasts traditional and more recent methods of teaching. You can find your own pictures on the internet to illustrate traditional methods of teaching medicine.

By the end of this short introduction you will have started to relate to your trainees and will have demonstrated good ways of interacting with them. Your trainees should be interested, immediately feel involved in the course, and be enjoying your style of training.

Aims

- To highlight key issues in teaching
- To get the message across in a way that demonstrates the best teaching methods.

Outline for the session

Time: 20 minutes

Resources: flip chart, pens, slides—pictures to show how medicine was taught in previous centuries

1. Introductory question
2. Trainer input
3. Task.

1 Introductory question

Ask the group whether they agree or disagree with the statement, 'I am a doctor, therefore I can teach'.

2 Trainer input

Picture contrasting traditional styles with recent developments using the visuals you have found. One picture might be a lecture theatre with the students sitting in banked rows and the professor directing doctors as they perform surgery on a patient.

3 Task

This task will encourage interaction right at the start of your course.

- Ask what characteristics they remember from their best teachers.
- Give trainees time to jot down the characteristics or qualities of a good teacher they have experienced.
- Encourage as many as possible to give one-word responses.

- Ask a scribe to write these up.
- Add any further ideas of your own, for example:
  patience
  love
  enthusiasm
  made us want to learn.
- Take a moment to reflect on the list. Many of the words will be about character and relationship rather than subject knowledge.

Remind your trainees of the central principle of relationship. Just as the nurse/ patient, doctor/ patient relationship is important, so the quality of the teacher/ student relationship will have a great impact on learning.

Additional material: names

Names are important. Aim to learn and use trainees' names by the end of the first day. This opening session is a good opportunity to start using names.
To achieve this:

- Read all the names before you start.
- Provide name badges that you can read from a distance.
- As trainees introduce themselves write down names on a seating plan.
- For the first day, encourage them to give their name whenever they speak.
- Take a photo of each one holding up their name badge so that you have a visual record to refer to at the end of the day.

Part 2

Before you teach: preparation and planning

Introduction to preparation and planning

Preparation means looking back as well as looking forward!

So much of the satisfaction of teaching well depends on the quality of your preparation. When you have thought carefully in advance about your teaching, you can approach it with confidence and enthusiasm. You have something important to say, and you have planned the best way of presenting it. Nevertheless, after you have taught, there will always be something that you will want to change. If you look back immediately after each session and reflect, you will realize what it is that you want to improve, for example you may have spent too long on a particular section or you may need some extra pictures. In fact you will never produce a perfect piece of teaching! Looking back and reflecting enables you to plan better for the next time you teach.

There is a great deal that you can anticipate. At first you do not know what some of these things are. Think for a moment about learning to drive. Learner drivers only focus on the car immediately in front, unable to take in pedestrians, bicycles, and a parked lorry 200 meters away. As they gain experience, they can avoid these dangers. In this section of the book, we want to help you anticipate pitfalls and prepare positively.

If you are teaching as part of an on-going programme then it is important that you follow the syllabus and cover what you are supposed to. Know the long-term goals of the curriculum or programme, and keep referring to them.

If you are building a new curriculum or series, then do not start with individual teaching sessions, but start by applying the initial six steps outlined in Chapter 2 to the whole body of teaching. (For more on curriculum review please turn to Appendix 3, page 193).

This part of the book is the longest because the quality of preparation determines the effectiveness and success of your teaching. Improve your preparation and you will improve your teaching.

Three key words to remember

Relationships

Relationships are at the heart of good teaching, because you, the teacher, affect what goes on in the heart and mind of the learner. If you build a good relationship, your students will respect you and want to learn from you. Inspiring teachers will have an impact on their student's career. Good relationships also offer the students freedom in their learning and personal development.

Teachers and students both have expectations of each other. You expect the learner to give you their attention, listen, participate, reflect, demonstrate learning, take notes, and do well in their examinations. Students expect clarity, structure, and a sense that you know what you are talking about and where you are going, and they need to trust what you teach.

Relevance

Everyone learns better if what they learn is directly relevant to them and their situation. Making the material relevant builds the relationship.

Responsibility

You are responsible for your students' learning. You are responsible for teaching them well. You are responsible in the first instance for finding solutions to any problems that occur in relation to teaching. What follows will help you fulfil this responsibility. Don't blame poor learning if you offer poorly prepared teaching.

CHAPTER 2

How to prepare efficiently: the essentials

Successful learning starts with good preparation. Good teaching does not just happen. It has been well prepared.

We will take you through six simple principles or steps and make some suggestions about choice of teaching method. We focus on timing and sorting out the room as part of essential preparation.

Your goal is to be an effective and inspiring teacher

What is effective teaching?

Teaching is effective when students:

- learn and remember what you teach
- gain knowledge, skills, or understanding
- enjoy learning and are inspired to learn more
- put into practice what they learn
- are motivated to learn by themselves.

What contributes most to effective teaching?

To find an answer, take a moment to think about a talk you have heard recently and which you can remember almost perfectly. What was it that helped you to remember it?

- the clear structure—you followed easily
- you understood what was important
- the enthusiasm of the speaker
- the concern of the speaker in helping you understand
- you understood everything
- the ability of the speaker to arouse your curiosity
- it was relevant to you
- it held your attention from start to finish
- there was good repetition to help you remember
- you were involved in different ways.

Every one of these points that helped you to remember was the result of good planning by the teacher. Every one of these points is something you can learn to do yourself and we will discuss them in Part 2. Planning well and preparing well contribute most to effective teaching.

Effective teaching does *not* depend on slides, good or bad, or on any technology—though you might choose to use it as a resource to enhance your teaching. Effective teaching starts with you, the teacher, thinking about what the students need to learn. Technology plays only a minor role in teaching.

We are going to look at six steps to follow every time you teach, when planning any type of teaching. Even if you use previous talks, there is always something to do differently. Do not use exactly the same talk for different audiences. You end up looking foolish when you have to skip slides that are not relevant. You do not have to start from scratch, but you do need to think about each teaching session and how best to present the material on that particular occasion.

Although these steps take a few pages to explain, you should be able to follow them in practice in a few minutes. In essence we are saying know your audience, your outcomes, your content, your location, and time available in advance. Choose your structure, the resources, and teaching method appropriately.

Six steps to preparation and planning

Step 1	**Who?**
Step 2	**Why?—aims**
Step 3	**What?—content**
Step 4	**How?—structure**
Step 5	**What else? Select and cut**
Step 6	**How to end?**

Step 1: Who? Thinking about the learners' needs

> Before you start working on content, stop and think about the students and how to make your material directly relevant to them.

Things to consider:

Audience—picture the audience and ask yourself some questions:

- What do they already know?
- What can they do well?
- What is their educational level (e.g. secondary school, college, degree, postgraduate)?
- What level are they professionally (e.g. experienced clinician)?
- How can I help them in the workplace and with their learning?
- Is my language their first language?*
- How must I adjust my own language to the audience if medical terminology is unfamiliar?

* Please refer to Appendix 1, page 183, if you need to think more about language issues. In the UK many students come from overseas and it may take them some time to understand everything you teach them.

Behaviour—theirs and mine

- How do I approach this group?
- How do I get them to pay attention?
- Do I need to check they understood a previous talk?
- Are they tired residents? Do I need to keep them awake?
- Are they a timid group? How will I draw out what they already know and encourage them?
- Are they a very lively group? How will I get them to focus on my teaching and not talking to each other? What shall I plan to do if they talk instead of listen?
- Is the group only focused on passing exams? How can I get them to think about their future work and application to patients?
- How prescriptive do I need to be? For example, if teaching a procedure in a medically unstable patient, do I need to be more rigid in what is safe for young students, or can I discuss options if talking to specialist trainees?

As you can see, questions about timing and time of day arise as soon as you begin to think about a particular teaching group, so you need to have in mind *now* your choice of teaching method.

Choice of method—how will I conduct the teaching?

- What will be the best method of delivery—interactive, tutorial, straight lecture, or a mix?
- What will the students do while I am talking? (see Hand-outs, page 34)

More detail on different methods or vehicles for delivering the content, are on page 16. Once you have an idea about method, carry on to the next step.

> A moment to focus clearly on who you are teaching will lead to more efficient planning.

Step 2: Why? Expressing clear aims

> Writing your aim will speed your preparation and give it focus. Clear aims are important. They enable you to clarify what you want your students learn. If you make your aims explicit, your students will know what they are supposed to learn and will concentrate on that.

Look at the topic and ask yourself:

- What is the most single important thing they need to know?
- What is the key take home message for this particular group?
- What change do I want to see in this group as a result of their learning?
  - *improved examination results*
  - *improved attitudes to patients*
  - *deeper understanding of problems, difficulties*
  - *ability to use a particular technique*
  - *willingness to search for more information*
  - *clearer thinking in solving problems*
  - *higher self esteem and the confidence to do all of the above.*

Such changes in behaviour are sometimes called learning outcomes. Answering these questions will help you to reach clear aims and write them down.

1. Express your aim in terms of what you want the learner to learn, the student's learning outcomes. Try not to think in terms of 'I am going to teach them anatomy today'. Rather, what they most need to remember and why.
   - what is the single most important error to avoid—and why?
   - what they should be able to do or understand or know at the end?

Try to avoid saying to more lowly groups, 'You don't need to know all of this'. Think how you are making the aims for your teaching appropriate to a specific group. For example:

In order to help the nurse to do a more responsible job:

- aim: to understand the beneficial effects of postoperative pain relief in children.

Here are some more examples:

That the students know/understand:

- the basic physiology so that ...
- when not to give a specific drug
- the benefits of talking to the patient
- the full range of options
- a clear list of causes.

2 Write down the aim/s for the teaching session that you will announce to your students. Make this explicit. If they too know where they are going, they are more likely to follow.

Your aim, their learning outcome, is the point to which your teaching is heading and everything in the teaching session must seek to achieve this.

Effective teaching sets out clear goals, and heads directly for them.

Step 3: What? Researching the content

Since you now have clear aims for specific learners, you can be selective in the sources you draw on, and select only what is appropriate to achieve the aim. You might start with your own knowledge, jotting down everything that comes into your head. Decide what is relevant to the topic and the learners.

Stand back from the content and think which areas are going to be hardest for your students. Give special attention to thinking how you will make these difficult things clear.

An example of what we mean is given in the box.

An example of thinking about the core content

Suppose you are teaching about fluid balance in small children—most people who are not paediatric specialists find this a difficult subject; they will easily understand and remember that the body composition is different in neonates, with a higher proportion of water in the body weight.

What are the areas where practitioners have difficulty, or may make serious mistakes? There are two:

(Contd.)

An example of thinking about the core content (*contd.*)

1. The need to assess and correct any existing deficit. The most common error is simply to 'apply the formula' which is a maintenance formula not a correction formula. Stress this point to prevent people making a serious mistake. Estimating the deficit requires:
   - history
   - clinical examination
   - possibly some investigations.
2. The difficulty in correctly remembering the maintenance formula—just to remind you, the 24-hour fluid requirements are:
   - 100ml/kg for the first 10 kg
   - 50 ml/kg for the next 10 kg
   - 20 ml/kg for all additional kg

Make sure the students:

- hear you say this
- see it written on a board, slide, or hand-out
- use it to calculate some examples for different sized children that you will supply.

Make sure the students understand that the above figures are *daily* requirements by getting them to calculate the corresponding *hourly* infusion rates. As an incentive to learn it, tell them that this knowledge will be tested later!

Keep up to date. Even if you are an expert in the field, check to see if any new information has been published. You cannot possibly cover everything on the topic and part of your responsibility is to select sources and direct your students to the best websites, journal articles, or textbooks for further information.

Planning the content and knowing what you want to teach comes before choice of methodology.

Step 4: How? The outline structure

A good structure helps the learner to organize the freshly acquired knowledge. Therefore it is easier to remember and retain.

Why is the structure important?

Developing your points in a clear fashion is crucial for clarity and for getting your message across. If you have a clear structure your students will remember what you say more easily. You need some section headings. If you think of your teaching as a journey, the subheadings are the stations along the route from the starting point to the end.

How will I structure my teaching?

Review your headings to ensure they relate to your aim.

Think about the order or sequence of each section. Re-order if necessary. You may well need to move the subheadings around until you are happy that you have the clearest route, the most logical order. Do this before you fill out the detail.

Only once you have a clear structure you can produce clear slides. Your slides are not your structure. (see Chapter 6, page 73 for hints on preparing slides). If you are not using slides, write up the headings as you go to reinforce the structure.

Sample structures

1 Use ABC or a mnemonic

ABC is obviously the key message in every talk on trauma management. It is repeated often and that is how we remember it. This only works in the English language. A Farsi-speaking group of trainees was asked to produce a poem with the equivalent words for Airway, Breathing, and Circulation in the correct order. They succeeded and now use this as an effective and culturally relevant way of remembering and teaching.

We used the letter R to emphasize the importance of three key words in the introduction to Part 2: relationship, responsibility, relevance.

2 Use questions, e.g. Why? What? How?

Structuring your sections around question words can be helpful for lectures, small group discussion and clinical demonstrations. It is also a way of involving the learners. Rhetorical or actual questions keep them listening and thinking.

It reflects the different ways we learn and includes all learning styles. We talk about this in greater depth in Chapter 12.

3 Use order and logic. If, for example, you are describing difficult airways, talk about nose, lips, tongue, teeth, jaw.

(Contd.)

Sample structures *(contd.)*

4 Use this outline for the presentation of a case study:
Introduction
Tell the story
Identify decisions that need to be made
Discuss consequences of different treatments
Get students to decide on treatment or management
Give reasons for your course of action
Reveal the actual outcome
Have a clear take home message, i.e. what you learnt from this case.

5 Follow the structure from a standard text book. After all, the authors have spent a lot of time writing and organizing the material.

Step 5: What else?

Do not try to tell your students everything *you* know.
Do not try to tell them everything there **is** to know.

Less is more. Most teaching is spoilt because there is too much of it! You will certainly have too much material. Far better to use your teaching time to focus on what is essential than to cram everything in. Keep each session lean.

- Select only that which takes your students towards your aim or learning outcomes. Keep reminding yourself what is really important and stick to it.
- Check that your sections are of equal length. Aim to keep your teaching moving at a sensible pace and cut out waffle, especially at the beginning, so that the first section is not too long.
- Read through what you are planning to do and then decide what else needs to be cut.
- Decide in advance what you will leave out if time runs out.

We cannot repeat often enough: less is more!

Step 6: And finally ... how to end!

Good planning includes planning to end well.

Ending well leaves your students with a clear take home message and a sense of a completed task.

We have all had too much material, spent too long on the opening section, rushed through the rest, and failed to repeat and summarize clearly. Inexperienced teachers fear not having enough material. That fear soon disappears.

- Decide the precise time when you must begin your summary or show your summary slide.
- Plan what you will drop if time runs out.
- Move to your summary at the time you planned, in order to finish on time.

This is important because it shows that you are in control of the time and your teaching. Those final moments are essential for repeating and reinforcing the main points you want everyone to remember.

Some teachers like to give their students time to look through their notes quietly before they leave. This is an excellent idea, but you must allow time for this. We suggest you give your students a few minutes at the end to think about what they have learned and to write down what they need to remember. Writing helps memory.

Some teachers like to allow a couple of minutes for people to ask for clarification if there is anything they have not understood. Beware of asking 'Any questions?' This can lead to a poor finish. (See Chapter 11 for more on taking questions.)

If you have introduced controversial material then *plan* to have a discussion. Allow time for this too. (See Chapter 4 for more on leading a discussion.)

At the end:

- Repeat what was most important
- Give your summary or put up a summary slide.

Send your students away with your message ringing in their ears, firmly planted in their brains.

Step	
Step 1	**Who?**
Step 2	**Why?—aims**
Step 3	**What?—content**
Step 4	**How?—structure**
Step 5	**What else? Select and cut**
Step 6	**How to end?**

Now you have taken these steps, what is left to prepare?

- the teaching method
- timing
- the room you will teach in.

Further refinements

In Chapter 3 we shall think about making a good start, maintaining attention, and preparing hand-outs. In Chapter 5 we deal in detail with preparation for an interactive session. In Chapter 6 we give hints on additional resources and visual aids. If you are going to use slides this should be a swift and easy task once you have the aims and structure of your talk.

Choosing the best teaching method

Whatever method you choose, whatever type of teaching you are doing (formal, informal, skill teaching), you need to follow the thinking about audience, aims, content, and structure because these areas of planning form the core or foundation of your preparation, from which everything else flows (Figure 2.1 below).

Time of day

Always consider the time of day when selecting your teaching method. A lecture necessarily packed full of facts will be more acceptable when students are fresh. It is to be avoided after lunch or at the end of a busy day. Try to pick a method that will require the active involvement of students just before and after lunch.

> Learn to experiment. Try different ways of teaching. Do not be afraid to mix methods whenever you feel it will be beneficial to your students.

WHO
are the learners
WHY
do they need
to learn this
WHAT
is the content
PREPARATION
FORMAL
LECTURE
MIXTURE OF
METHODS
CASE STUDY
SKILL
TEACHING
INTERACTIVE
SEMMINAR

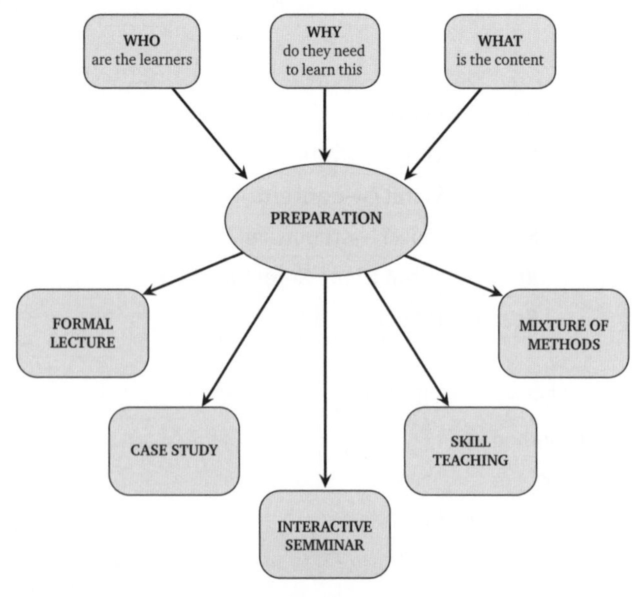

Figure 2.1

The formal lecture

This is most suitable for large groups numbering more than 30. It is the normal method of presenting at conferences and meetings. This traditional method allows the teacher to present and teach what they have prepared without active participation. The formal lecture is a good way of conveying a large amount of factual knowledge. The greatest danger is to assume that because you have given your lecture, others will have heard and remembered it!

In the next chapter we give advice on gaining and maintaining attention for ensuring the best ways for students learn from a lecture.

Remember that this format need not exclude interactive elements!

An interactive teaching method

This involves interactions between the students and the teacher. The teacher still has to prepare and know where the session is going. It is most suitable for groups of up to a maximum of 30.

Using questions and answers is ideal to consolidate, revise, and build on what is already known. It is less suitable for introducing a new topic.

If you are serious about wanting to improve your teaching, then you need to move away from the traditional lecture to interactive teaching. This style of teaching is so important that in Chapter 5 we go into this in great detail. In that chapter we tell you how to approach this method to gain the skills you need, and how to prepare.

A mix of methods

The formal lecture and a question and answer session are not mutually exclusive. You can introduce interactive elements into a formal lecture. You can use questions interactively at the start of a more formal lecture and then continue with fewer interactions. You can begin formally and find ways of letting students learn interactively during the lecture. When you prepare, always think about how to involve the students in what you are teaching. You will find more ideas for bringing variation into a formal lecture in Chapter 3.

Teaching through case studies

This is an enjoyable method which we use for almost any group of learners. It is ideal for groups of up to 30. It involves you choosing a specific case from your own experience, which is a good vehicle for conveying specific teaching points. The structure outlined on page 16 demonstrates that interactions with the learners are built in to this method. We devote Chapter 4 to this type of teaching.

A tutorial

This method of teaching can be led by either the teacher or by one or more students who will need to prepare carefully. It is most suitable for groups of up to 12.

There is a great advantage in your being able to assess the students' knowledge and their ability to communicate it. The other advantage is that the students do more work than you, although you do still need to think in advance about the points they should be covering. In our experience, you have to be very firm about the fact that the student is going to prepare, and clear about your expectations. You should direct them to useful sources of information. Tell them to avoid trawling the internet uncritically.

A debate

This is excellent for approaching controversial aspects of medicine and can be adapted for quite large groups. It is important to choose two people on each side of a debate who will put a point of view with some clear reasons. After two speakers for and against the issue, others should be encouraged to express their view. This is a good way to prepare students for an essay on moral issues. It can be a difficult method for those taught by traditional and authoritarian professors.

We are not including any material on problem-based learning as this is beyond the scope of this book, which is not aimed at the structure of learning in university medical schools.

Getting the timing right

Why is timing important?

Timing is important as it shows you are thinking of your teaching group and also being considerate to the next lecturer or the people the students are going off to work with next. If you ignore the time and overrun nobody in your audience will be listening. They will all be thinking about getting home or getting in the coffee queue—so there is no point overrunning.

Experienced teachers know exactly what they can fit comfortably into a teaching session. They know that you can plan your timing.

How can I get the timing right?

1 When giving a talk:
   - (i) Know before you start how long you have and the precise finishing time.
   - (ii) Work out how long you plan to spend on each section. Be aware if you are overrunning on the first section.
   - (iii) Write down approximate timings on your teaching plan or slide printout in advance.
   - (iv) Decide what you can leave out if time goes.
   - (v) Allow adequate time for reflection, reading of hand-outs, or possible questions before you round everything off with the main take-home message.
   - (vi) Just before you start, put your watch where you can see it.
   - (vii) If you practise at home, you must accept and remember that the actual teaching needs about 10 minutes per hour longer than the practice.

(viii) Be prepared to be flexible. Most teaching starts a few minutes late. When that happens, do not rush. You have prepared in advance the bit you will omit.

(ix) Ask a friend to indicate when you have 5 minutes then 1 minute left.

2 When organizing groups and workshops:

(i) Work out in advance how long you will need for group tasks. Do not forget to include time for people to move.

(ii) If you are organizing rotating groups, keep an eye on the clock and give everyone equal time. Tell them how long they will have.

(iii) When running a series of small group tasks, give a 5-minute warning before they end.

(iv) If you are teaching a new skill, give everyone the chance to have a turn. Allow time for the students to help you tidy up. Then give time for them to discuss what they have achieved.

Preparing the room

This is the final task before you stand up and teach.

Take control of your space

You are responsible for your teaching environment. This means getting there in good time before you start not only to get any slides ready but also to see the layout of the room. If you are not in a lecture theatre, you may well want to rearrange the seating. If you are in a large lecture theatre with only a few people present and they sit at the back, you can ask them to come and fill up the front rows.

Now consider the temperature of the room. Do you need to open windows or turn up the heating so that everyone will be more comfortable? Think about all these things when you visit your teaching room before you teach.

Plan your seating

Think about the teaching method you have chosen. What different arrangements can you have?

- For a formal lecture you will probably have little opportunity to make changes to the room. However, even if you are in a small space with large tables you can try a couple of alternatives. One way is to have the tables in a large block (Figure 2.2a, overleaf). If you start formally you can then move to a more informal setting for teaching interactively.

  The other way is to have the students facing you in rows (Figure 2.2b, overleaf). This can be a good way to end the day, changing the tables to a more formal setting to indicate that the final section of teaching is serious.

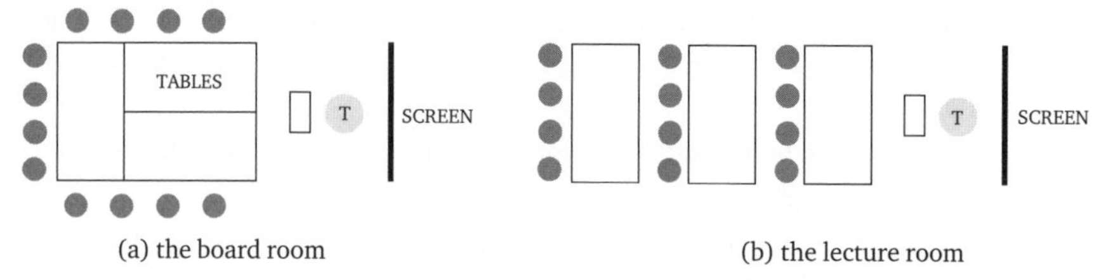

(a) the board room (b) the lecture room

Figure 2.2 Seating for formal teaching.

- When you plan to teach interactively you want to be able to approach the students and have room to move. A horseshoe arrangement opens up the room and indicates that something different is about to happen (Figure 2.3).

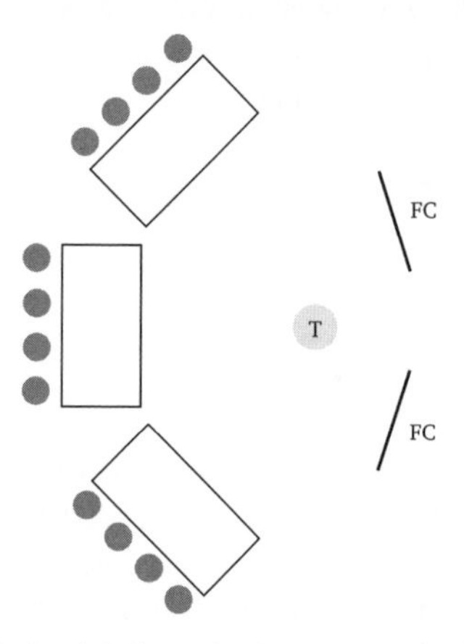

Figure 2.3 Seating for easier interaction: the horseshoe.

- When you anticipate getting your students to work in small groups, think where you want them to work. You may need to move tables apart (or ask them to do this), or you may need to ask everyone to move their chairs, so that they end up in groups as you had planned (Figure 2.4). They must be able to hear each other and talk easily, even if they have to sit around fixed tables. Always glance around to make sure that nobody appears to be excluded from the discussion.

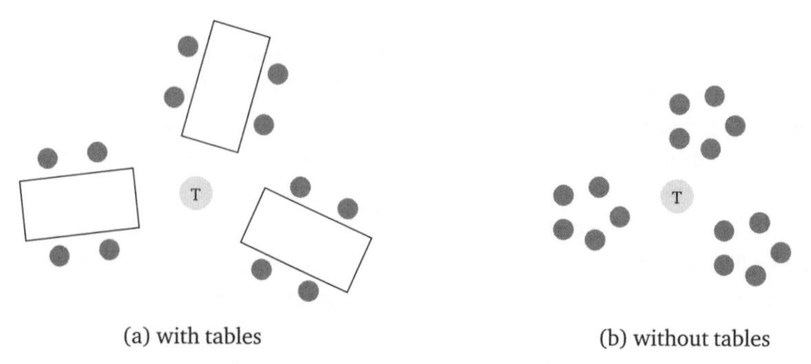

(a) with tables (b) without tables

Figure 2.4 Seating for informal, small groups.

The simplest arrangement is to have a circle of chairs for an informal teaching session (Figure 2.5).

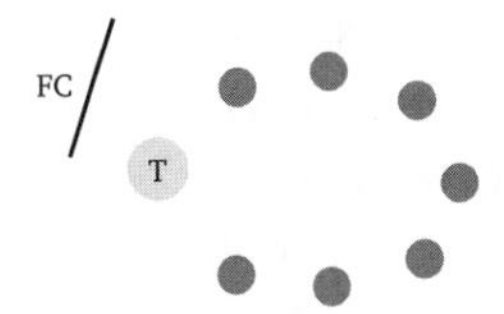

Figure 2.5 Seating for informal discussion with the teacher.

- Why bother with this? Have you ever changed the layout of the room? The way the room is laid out affects the atmosphere. Changing the atmosphere and moving people around affects relationships. It helps a new group get to know each other. Think about the best arrangement for pair work, or discussion.
- If nothing in the room can be moved, you at least can change your position. You can stand at the back behind the class when you show slides. Getting students to interact in pairs is always possible.

Check the position of any resources

Put out hand-outs and get any equipment ready.

Using slides:

When you visit the room you should not only check the projection equipment, but also the blackout, and position of the large screen.

See where the small table is placed for your laptop.

Plan your use of the flip chart:

What will I write on? Is there enough fresh paper?

Where are the pens? Do the pens work?

Do I need to write up any headings?

Do I need to get the outline drawn for a diagram?

Do I need to move it so that everyone can see?

Using a board:

Check that you have non-permanent pens for the whiteboard. Do they write?

Check that there is chalk if you planned to use a chalk board.

Is there a board wiper? If not collect some damp paper towels from the nearest washroom.

Take charge of your learning environment and get it ready, as you want it, before the students arrive.

When you leave, try to leave it as you found it or would like to find it. Clear the board. Put tops on felt tip writers. Return the furniture to its normal position.

Time to stop and think

- Do I need to rethink how I plan for teaching?
- When am I going to try out the six steps?
- When is the best time to start teaching more interactively?
- How am I going to improve my timing?
- Can I make better use of the room by planning a different arrangement?

Notes for Trainers

How to prepare efficiently—the essentials

Successful learning starts with good preparation on the part of the teacher. Good teaching does not just happen. It has been well prepared and planned.

Aims

- To define the basic steps necessary for good teaching
- To encourage trainees to be more creative in all aspects of planning for teaching.

Outline for the session: the basics of preparation

Time: 60–90 minutes
Resources: slides, hand-out, outlines for task, Oxford Handbook
Sample hand-out: Appendix 4, Hand-out 1

1. Introductory remarks
2. Trainer input: the six steps to good planning (10–20 minutes depending on detail)

Additional material: memory and learning

3. Tasks on setting aims
4. Different teaching methods
5. Timing and finishing
6. Time to reflect

Additional material: preparing the room
Sample slide set.

1 Introductory remarks

Ask your trainees what they think is proof of a successful course. Collect their responses then show the bullet points as slides. You might ask if the trainees consider themselves to be willing learners.

Give them three key words, which are going to return throughout the course: relationships, responsibility, and relevance.

Explain that planning and preparation are essential for every type of teaching: the lecture, the interactive seminar, the discussion group, teaching a skill. (How to decide on the most suitable method: see page 20.)

2 Trainer input: the six steps to good planning

Keep stressing that good teaching doesn't just happen. Move through the six steps fairly fast. There is a sample slide set of this. Prepare these six steps on slides and repeat each principle as you finish each slide.

Prepare a summary slide in which the trainees repeat each named step and then you display that point.

Continue to point out that all of this preparation happens before you think about preparing any slides.

Here are some further questions to consider for Step 1 when planning for a specific group of learners:

- Which aspects of their practice, knowledge base, or understanding need to improve the most?
- Who are the patients who present to this group?
- What equipment is available to them?
- Which patients should they never treat?
- Do you need to go back a step and revise some physiology and basic science?
- What drugs or treatment is available?
- How difficult is it for this group to change their normal practice? If I am giving a new way of doing something, how will I get them to accept change and put it into practice?
- How will I approach a group that never seems interested?

When you talk about clarity of purpose, knowing what your aims are, communicating them clearly you must not only continually emphasize this but also demonstrate it in your presentations and input.

You must set out clear aims for each of your sessions and have prepared a good summary slide.

Additional material: memory and learning

For a longer course here is an aside on memory and learning. We want our students to remember what we teach.

What is easier: to recall a fact or to recognize which of two facts is correct? If I ask you to give me the word in a foreign language for a pink spring flower, it is difficult to recall. If I offer two alternatives, e.g. hyacinth or daffodil, then you recognize the correct word. It is essential for you to recall a huge amount of information. This information must be stored in the long-term memory. It must be easily accessed. For easy access we need to organize or structure what we teach. For example if you have a random list of names of nerves, they will be difficult to recall. If the names are presented in a structured way and grouped under headings, that will mean quicker retrieval from the long-term memory.

If students are going to remember what we teach, we need to:

- organize our teaching material very clearly
- repeat key points
- use mnemonics.

3 Tasks on setting aims

TASK 1: WRITING APPROPRIATE AIMS

15 minutes

- Choose a teaching topic relevant to your trainees and a group that they will teach, e.g. residents, nurses.
- Write up the name of the topic and ask your trainees on their own to write aims for that session. They should express their aims in terms of what the students should know or be able to do at the end of the teaching.
- Change the nature of the student group that they will teach and ask your trainees to adapt their aims.
- Allow each trainee to compare their aims with one other person.
- Ask one or two pairs to read their preferred aims and write these up.

TASK 2: INDIVIDUAL PREPARATION LEADING TO A GROUP DISCUSSION

- Choose three or four topics from your Oxford Handbook. Give the page reference for these topics to different groups, who must imagine they are going to teach the topic to new specialist residents.

Private study 20–30 minutes

- On their own each trainee should prepare:
    1. aims
    2. headings for a clear outline structure
    3. a summary slide.

Group workshop 20–30 minutes

- Each group assigned the same topic meets with a trainer. The group shares their aims, structure, and summaries. Through discussion they arrive at the best set of aims, structure, and summary, which they record onto flip chart paper.

Reporting back 10 minutes

- The whole class reassembles and a representative from each group reports back.

This task gives opportunity for good discussion, practice at writing legibly, presenting group findings, and provides some good teaching resources for future use.

TASK 3: ADVANCED PLANNING USING JOURNAL ARTICLES

Give your students an article from a reputable journal relevant to their speciality:

- Allow enough time to read it and take it in.
- Tell them to imagine they have to present the article. Give advice on presenting the arguments in the article. Take time to discuss and agree the main points.
- Divide your trainees into small groups of two or three. Give groups different target audiences, e.g. medical students, residents, a presentation to consultants.
- Ask them to write the most important message they think that their target group should understand from their review of the article.
- Ask a representative of each type of audience to feedback before further discussion.

A variation in their small groups; they discuss how they would word their aim if presenting the article to a group of medical students. Then everyone decides how it would change if presenting the content of the article to a departmental meeting.

4 Different teaching methods

Try to present this material interactively. Most trainees will come up with most of it themselves.

5 Timing and finishing

Talk with the whole group about why this is important. Try to include contributions from as many as possible.

6 Time to reflect

Set a pattern of reflecting and noting down what they want to remember. Make sure you leave time to do this in a calm manner.

Additional material: preparing the room

Do make sure you keep your teaching room tidy. If possible, change the seating before this session. Try to ensure a fresh look after lunch!

If you are doing a longer course, you might include these practical considerations either at the end of planning or after the section on brainstorming. If you are teaching a short course, include them after the whole interactive teaching section.

Slide set for six steps to successful preparation

Students are learning
Students enjoy learning
Students want to learn more

Planning your teaching Step 1

Take time to think about your learners

- Who are they?
- What do they already know?
- What is their level?
- How can I make this relevant to *this* group?

Step 1: Who?

Planning your teaching Step 2

Write a clear aim for your teaching

- If concepts: that they should understand…
- If facts: that they should learn and know…
- If skills: that they should be able to …

Step 2: Why?

Why is this important?

Planning your teaching Step 3

Research and gather your material

Step 3: What?

Gathering the content

Planning your teaching Step 4

Plan a clear structure

- Get simple headings
- Relate headings to aims
- Think about order of headings

Step 4: How?

How do I structure the material?

Planning your teaching Step 5

Select and cut—*less is more*

- Do not try to tell them everything you know!
- Do not tell them everything there is to know!

Step 5: What else must I do?

What should I cut out?

Planning your teaching Step 6

Plan how you will end!

- Write your summary
- What was most important? Repeat this
- Plan what *time* you start your summary
- Plan what you will omit if time runs out

Step 6: How?

How am I going to finish?

Planning your teaching

Refinements

- Starting well
- Keeping attention
- Pace and timing
- Resources: equipment, visuals
- What are the students doing?

Planning your teaching six steps: Summary

1 Who? Think about the learner
2 Why Is this important? Write aims
3 What? Gather the content
4 How? Find a good structure
5 What else? What should I cut out?
6 How will I finish?

CHAPTER 3

How to prepare for a formal lecture: keeping your students interested and alert

> Gaining and maintaining the attention of students is the responsibility of the teacher.

Introduction

Let us assume you have to give a formal lecture and you have prepared as far as the aims, structure, and main content. You may not yet be satisfied with what you have. In this chapter we are going to tell you about some of the refinements that turn an ordinary lecture into one that people remember. We shall focus on getting a good start, which is of course relevant to all teaching, and then think about how to hold the attention of a group for longer than 20 minutes. After considering what stops some students from concentrating, we have some ideas for hand-outs, which you can use as another way of maintaining attention.

How to start: ways of gaining attention

RELEVANCE

The best way to engage your audience from the outset is to make the teaching directly relevant to them. Develop a repertoire of new ways of gaining interest, extras which will help them remember. Become a creative teacher!

Here are some ideas:

- Ask if anyone has had experience of the topic you will be teaching.
- Set a real, local context and tell it as a story. You can refer to an event or patient on a ward or in the operating room last week. This makes the topic immediate. They will know this could occur any time in their daily practice.
- Find a way of telling them why it is important. Be personal and tell them how it is relevant in your life, or why you find it interesting.
- If they are sleepy, wake them up, get them to stand up, open some windows. Yours may be the third lecture in a row.
- Try a surprise at the start—a relevant but interesting picture, a question, or perhaps video clip with sound. Perhaps you have a cartoon to show.
- Prediction is a good way of gaining and keeping attention. Ask the students to write in advance what they think they need to know on the subject: ask them to write down the problems they could expect; ask them to write down what they most want to learn from the lecture, or do not understand about the topic. This way they will listen to see if you cover these. If you do not address what worries them, then there will be genuine questions at the end.
- Even with a traditional lecture you can begin with a question or puzzle which they discuss in pairs before you start.
- Bring in a piece of equipment linked to your topic and ask a question about it.
- Use a suggestion from Chapter 5, page 51 about how to start with a question to brainstorm what should already be known.

There is a further benefit of arousing curiosity at the start. We want people to remember what we teach. To store information in the long-term memory we need to open up the pathways to the brain. One way of doing this is to make people curious. If you are used to hearing good preaching, you will know that the preacher often starts with an anecdote or funny story. It is not just to amuse you. It is to engage your attention and will help you to remember all that follows.

Holding attention and varying the stimulus

It is your responsibility to keep everyone's attention for the whole lecture. You can and must plan for this too! If you have thought about and carefully selected the content, then all of it is important. You want everyone to follow for the entire session.

HOW ARE YOU GOING TO KEEP THE STUDENTS ALERT AND INTERESTED?

Most people can concentrate for 20 minutes. Know when you are 20–25 minutes in to your teaching and *be prepared* for the concentration dip!

There are ways of telling when concentration begins to fall off. Learn to be aware of the responses of your audience. Notice if eyes are closing; notice if what is outside the window is more interesting than what you are saying; notice if people start writing or talking, looking at watches, or just looking bored.

When you notice that the audience is drifting, what can you do to get them back? Do something different, vary the stimulus! Here are some ideas:

- Switch off your slides and ask what was on the screen.
- Use the <B> or <W> key (see Chapter 8, page 104), move away from the slides and
  - *tell a story*
  - *ask a question and give them time to talk about the answer together.*
- Ask them to stand up and turn around.
- Introduce a picture or moving pictures.
- Stop talking and give them something to read. Perhaps hand out a photocopy of a relevant journal article and give time to read it and find the answer to a question.
- Stop talking after asking a rhetorical question, and give everyone a moment to think.

Here are some further ideas to vary the stimulus:

- Direct attention to a piece of equipment and ask a question related to it.
- Ask for a volunteer to demonstrate.
- Get the students to read a relevant section from a text book, then explain the difficult bit or illustrate with examples from your practice.
- Use a flip chart for a quick diagram.
- Keep bringing the material back to the interests of the audience and perhaps get a show of hands on a point where opinion might differ.

You are responsible for gaining and keeping the attention of your audience. If they stop listening, you must try to make them listen: vary the stimulus! Even in the most formal conference address, you can try a change of visual or change of pace after 20 minutes, or if you are speaking for an hour, do this again after 40 minutes. Plan carefully the points at which you need to vary what you are doing.

Barriers to learning

In spite of all your best efforts, there will be times when people simply cannot concentrate. You need to be aware of this. Some of the barriers to learning can be overcome if you establish interest at the beginning. What can you do about any of these?

EXTERNAL BARRIERS

- Extraneous noise: distractions such as mobile phones and texting; colleagues tapping away on their computers; noise of traffic; people outside the room; what is going on outside the window; building work.
  You can certainly do something about mobile phones. Ban them. Issue an ultimatum to younger students that they either text outside or turn them off and remain in the class.
  Dealing with more senior colleagues and those on call is trickier. Accept the situation will not be perfect. You may think about seating the person who continues

to use his laptop throughout your lecture at the back of the room. Allocate a table with a nearby source of electricity!
- Weather: bright sunlight, thunderstorms, gathering darkness and not knowing when you will finish.

Make sure you always finish on time.

- Physical discomfort: hunger, thirst, heat, cold, hard chairs.
Be aware of these difficulties. You can do something about many of them. Prepare the room, allow them to stand up at some point, allow them to have a short snack midway. In some countries students leave home extremely early to get to the hospital and will not have had breakfast. Better to agree a 5-minute delayed start, and have them refreshed than sitting feeling faint for an hour.

INTERNAL BARRIERS

- Anxiety: relationship problems, money problems, worry about illness—their own or a relative's.
You have to be more interesting than the problem! They have to know that what you are about to teach is of greater importance at that moment.
- Perceived threat: having to answer a question, ignorance and losing face, speaking next in public.
These may not relate to teaching in a lecture unless you have a tendency to throw out an unexpected question and pick on someone to answer. Avoid doing that.
- Dislike of you the teacher because of gender attitudes, perceived superiority, lack of interest in the group.
This can be overcome to some extent by making the content relevant and showing interest in the learning needs of the students. Just being aware of their levels of discomfort in the room and doing something will increase their appreciation of what you are teaching. You should not aim to be liked, but you can expect to be respected for the quality of your teaching.

Any of these physical or emotional barriers will effectively stop students hearing what you are saying. All of these are good reasons why you need to have well-prepared material. But there are times when people need your sympathy and you must be flexible and realistic about what you will achieve on a given day.

Planning hand-outs

Hand-outs can be of great help so plan in advance why, when, and how you want to use them. They can give students a focus while you lecture.

DO YOU NEED A HAND-OUT?

Hand-outs can be a helpful way of reinforcing your lecture and keeping the students interested. A hand-out gives a counter-focus to any source of distraction. Photocopying may be expensive and takes time, but used sparingly hand-outs are an important source of support for students' learning.

Avoid giving the students a full hand-out of your notes or slides at the start. Everyone will skim through when you start talking. They will miss what you are saying while not really concentrating on what you have written.

WHEN WILL YOU WANT TO USE HAND-OUTS?

Give out a hand-out at the *beginning* if you have:

- a diagram you want them to label
- a problem you want them to discuss and write down answers
- complex formulae that need to be accurate and worked on
- a list of new medical terminology you will refer to
- a clear structure and you want the students to fill in the detail
- relevant MCQs
- a revision question.

Give out a hand-out in the *middle* if you have explained complex matters and wish to give them all time to read in silence to see if everyone has understood. A hand-out varies the stimulus.

Give out a hand-out at the *end* in order to:

- give time to read everything before they leave
- apply their new knowledge by solving a problem case
- do a set of MCQs
- to write down what they have learned under your headings
- set out what needs to be done next, or extra sources of information.

WHAT HAPPENS WHEN YOU USE HAND-OUTS IN THESE WAYS?

The students will be:

- thinking because you have set some preliminary questions
- using their imaginations and learning predictive skills; if you explain the context and give a good case history, they can write down how they think the management of the patient proceeded
- working things out, if you present your material with a problem to solve
- listening carefully, if you give them some opening questions that you expect them to be able to answer when you finish teaching
- reading, if you give them time within your teaching
- writing detail, if you give them a gapped hand-out with only your headings

- writing questions, if you ask them at the beginning to jot down what they do not understand.

Hand-outs should be a tool to help students learn actively.

Being creative

> Develop a wide repertoire of ways of starting, maintaining attention, and finishing. Collect new ideas for your teaching. Be a risk taker and try a new method.

Are you beginning to get the picture that teaching is relational—it is an interaction between people? It begins with you thinking about the needs of the students. Your attitude to them is what will make the greatest difference to your teaching. If you rush in late, grumpy and resentful from a meeting or the operating theatre, nobody will enjoy it. Even 5 minutes' thought given to your aim, structure of key points, and what they should do and/or know at the end will make a huge difference. Without your students' engagement, your teaching will be ineffective. Follow the six steps we outlined, go the extra mile in making material relevant and varied, and you will be well on the way to being effective.

More than this, teaching is a way of being innovative. You should have fun when you are teaching and enjoy the process itself. Be bold and try out ideas. Start to work through the refinements. Copy good ideas from other people and make them part of your repertoire. If you take this approach to your preparation you will find it transforms your teaching.

What if it goes wrong?

Do not be afraid to admit to yourself that some teaching did not go well. It happens. You can use such an occasion as a spur to reflect on why it did not go well. Was it was lack of preparation, a poor structure, too much content, poor explanations, lack of a hand-out, a poor start, poor time-keeping? Having analysed the problem, enjoy turning this situation around and be creative in preparing for the next. Try some student interactions, a different way of dividing the group, a different structure. Above all, become a creative teacher.

Be a creative teacher, learn from your mistakes.

Time to stop and think

- How can I make things more relevant?
- Do I ever think about how I keep the attention of the group for the whole lecture?
- What ideas do I want to try out?
- Am I sympathetic to sources of discomfort? Do I do anything to break down barriers to learning?
- When am I going to plan a useful hand-out? How and when will I use it?

Notes for Trainers

How to prepare for a formal lecture

A good teacher needs to build a large repertoire of different ways to help students remember. You must keep students awake, interested, and help them to organize their knowledge.
This is the message that you, the trainer, must keep repeating.

Aims

- To increase ability to give a good lecture or seminar
- To help understand why the involvement of learners is important
- To encourage creativity in teaching.

Outline for the session: further aspects of planning

Time: 60–90 minutes
Resources: slides, outlines for task, Oxford Handbook
Sample hand-out: Appendix 4 Hand-out 1

1. Introduction
2. Trainer input:
    - Gaining attention—relevance
    - Maintaining attention—surviving the concentration dip
    - Barriers to learning
    - Hand-outs
3. Tasks
4. Time to reflect.

1 Introduction

Show your own aims to give security to your audience

Gaining attention and getting off to a good start is essential. You must demonstrate this!

Begin by revising the six steps for good preparation.

What has the trainee already done by way of preparation?

- thought about the audience
- written aims
- researched the content
- produced a clear structure
- cut
- written a summary.

Some ideas for you, the trainer, to gain attention:

Use a question-starter to get people thinking about their answer, then display your answer. Some examples:

- *Anyone* can teach?
  No! Anyone can *learn* to teach.
- My aim is to get through to the coffee break?
- My aim is to get to the end of my lecture?
  No! My aim is to enable the students to learn something.

2 Trainer input

Give an outline of what you will cover:

- time of day
- gaining attention—relevance
- memory—if you have not yet talked about memory, do this now (Chapter 2, page 29 *Additional material*)
- maintaining attention—surviving the concentration dip
- barriers to learning
- hand-outs.

Explain why these points are necessary, that the trainees are now operating on a number of levels. When they give a lecture they are using equipment/ slides; keeping an eye on the time; and assessing the response of the learners. This is multi-tasking in a big way. And there is more to think about…

Approach the sections in different ways so that you avoid giving a series of lists.

- Use slides to list for ideas for relevance. Act them out as you go through them.
- Give out a hand-out before starting to talk about maintaining attention. Tell a story after 20 minutes and then point out that they had hit the concentration dip!
- Gather ideas for barriers to learning interactively. Write headings in advance on the flip chart.
- Ask the class in pairs to think about an idea for using hand-outs at different stages of a lecture, then give your ideas.

Once you finish your input, you want the trainees to apply new ideas immediately.

3 Tasks to apply the principles of gaining and maintaining attention

TASK 1: IMPROVING A BORING SLIDE LECTURE

- Ask a trainer to read a printout of a well-structured lecture in a very boring manner. Their words should be exactly the same as text slides on the screen.
- While this dull lecture is being given, trainees make notes on the following:
  what is good about the preparation, e.g. structure
  how to improve it, e.g. through relevance to the specific audience
  interactions: jot down questions that could have been asked
  when to use the flip chart or the <B> or <W> key (see page 106)
  what else does this talk need?
- Trainees discuss in pairs advice on how to turn this into a successful teaching session.
- Feedback should focus on sharing the most important improvement from each pair.

TASK 2: GAINING ATTENTION!

15–20 minutes

- Choose the appropriate number of topics from the Oxford Handbook.
- Divide trainees into pairs. Two sets of pairs are given the same topic.
- Each pair must work completely separately from the other pair to produce the following outline on paper (Points 1–5) as if they were preparing to teach the topic for 20–30 minutes:
  1. aims, i.e. what you want students to know, recognize, or be able to do at the end
  2. a statement explaining why this is important
  3. a structured plan, with headings only
  4. a summary slide
  5. most importantly, they take time to find a way of making the introduction interesting, grabbing attention, and rousing curiosity. They write down their idea for gaining interest.

10 minutes

- Pairs with the same topic come together and exchange plans, which they read carefully and critically.
- As a group of four, they discuss what they learned from each other, especially noting ideas for gaining attention (Point 5).

- One person from each pair reports back to the whole group their best idea for gaining attention.
- By the end, the group should have a good list of various ideas to try out.

4 Time to reflect

Now is a good time to ask the trainees to finish by writing down all their ideas on the section of Hand-out 1, Ideas, which you may have used when introducing the topic of preparation.

CHAPTER 4

How to prepare case studies for teaching

INTRODUCTION

Case studies are an excellent vehicle for clinical teaching and are now increasingly used to provoke discussion and debate. We teach with case studies to present a wide range of interesting current practice and to demonstrate ways of interactive teaching, which are a clear departure from traditional methods. You may have been using them for years but do follow this chapter to see if there are aspects of your case presentations that you could improve.

WHAT DO WE MEAN BY CASE PRESENTATION?

A case presentation is a way of teaching as if you had the actual patient with you. It is an excellent way of focusing clinical teaching. It combines realism with the interest of telling a story. The students have time to reflect on the significance of the information, and are able to compare their ideas and expectations with the actual outcome. Presenting a case can be a way of intriguing your students, raising curiosity, and maintaining their interest as you reveal additional features of the clinical story in stages. As the case unfolds, they become involved in learning and understanding important facts step by step—rather like a good murder mystery!

Selecting and structuring the case presentation

HOW DO YOU CHOOSE A GOOD CASE TO TEACH FROM?

1. Have a real case. Audiences will easily identify a case that you have invented; the sense of reality immediately disappears, and they lose interest in the outcome. The best cases are the ones drawn from your own personal experience.

2 Choose a case that illustrates the message you want to get across. Think about the points you want to make and select a suitable case, rather than picking a case because you did something clever.
3 Consider a case in which you had a problem, a clear choice of procedures, or one in which something unexpected turned up. This moment of decision or crisis will open up discussion during the presentation.
4 Remember to choose a case which is relevant to the group you are teaching.

HAVING CHOSEN THE CASE, FOLLOW THE NORMAL STEPS OF PREPARATION

Like any other teaching session, you need to prepare and plan. There is excellent scope for interactive teaching, and because the students will remember the story, they have a framework for also remembering the teaching points.

- Clear aim.
  Keep it simple so that your message comes across strongly and clearly—so don't pick 'the most difficult case I have ever encountered'.
  Prepare clear teaching aims, just as you would for any other teaching session.
- Clear structure. This includes:
  introduction, setting the scene
  telling the story, introducing the patient to the group
  planning your questions, asking for opinions and providing any further information they may need
  giving more information, asking them to interpret it
  identifying what decisions have to be made
  discussing the consequences of different treatment options
  getting the class to decide (on the diagnosis, management, or both)
  revealing the outcome
  applying the lessons to their own experience and practice.
- Select and cut. Remove personal details. It should not be possible to identify the patient so if, for example, you include copies of lab results, make sure the name is blanked out. Avoid photographs that would allow the patient to be identified. Remember you are not going to tell your students everything there is to know about the subject. You have to decide what is important and stick to that.
- Clear summary. Even if the case appears complex, the 'take-home' message should be clear and simple.
- Work on the detail:
  plan your questions and interactions (this is so important that we devote Chapter 5 to explaining how to do this)
  plan how you will tell the story
  plan the discussion which you will lead afterwards
  plan slides and other resources.

Here are some points specific to preparing a case presentation:

- Scan in the actual paperwork. Highlight the detail on the real documents. Do remember to remove any personal details of the patient.
- Prepare selected detail of results and investigations.
- Do *not* give all the biodetail of the patient. That is part of the story you tell.
- Do *not* make slides of the whole narrative.

Please read Chapter 6, pages 73 on how to prepare helpful slides.

An example of how to plan a case study

- Introduce the case with a general comment suggesting why the material is important, e.g.

  'There are 600,000 maternal deaths in the world each year...'

  'The incidence of drug-resistant tuberculosis increases by 30% each year...'

  'Surveys show that 17.5 million British adults complain of backache...'

  This tells the students what area you are going to deal with, and why it's important. This can also be done in the case of a rare condition: *'Although Reye's syndrome affects only about 500 patients a year in the US, it is vital to recognize it because the fatality rate may be as high as 50%, and this is reduced by early diagnosis'.*
- Introduce us to the patient. Avoid doing this by putting all the patient's biodata on a slide. Tell the history as it was received, with the usual mixture of clear clues, hints, and things that were irrelevant. You are not a writer of fiction, so your aim is not to deceive the audience, or hold back information that may later prove to be critical. If you are presenting to a specialist audience you may also want to give specialist history, e.g. *'Mrs Kumar* comes to your clinic complaining of breathing problems. She has *an obstetric history of three pregnancies, with two miscarriages and one premature birth at 23 weeks of a baby who died'.*
- Now is a good time for some interaction:

  Open question:

  'What do you think the cause of her symptoms might be?'

  Closed question:

  'Write down the three most likely reasons for her breathlessness.'

(Contd.)

An example of how to plan a case study (*contd.*)

Follow up with:

'What further questions would you ask the patient?'

'When you examine the patient, what would you be looking for?'

'What further tests might be helpful?'

You must provide the answers to any questions from the students at this stage. This is one key reason why you should have a 'real' case of which you have personal knowledge.

- At this stage you could give some further information and guidance, for example you could summarize:

  'So we have a pregnant lady with unexplained breathlessness. It's important to confirm or rule out thromboembolic disease here, and to think about what predisposing causes she might have.'

  Caution! Someone in the class will by now have spotted that the patient has factor V Leiden syndrome. You may want to let that come out, but if your main teaching point is 'how to make the diagnosis of pulmonary embolism (PE)', it is easy to get sidetracked here. To avoid getting sidetracked, you might say 'Some of you may have an idea about a predisposing cause for these symptoms, but what we need to do first is to think about how we would confirm the diagnosis of PE. Let's have a show of hands; if you could only do one investigation, which of these would it be?'

  chest radiograph

  ECG

  V/Q scan

  MRI of lungs.

  Ask someone who voted for the correct answer why they did so. Then show the class the results of the investigation and ask them to report and interpret it.

- Display some actual results. If the results you show confirm the diagnosis of PE, ask whether that makes the diagnosis certain. What would be the rationale for treating even if the diagnosis was not certain? What treatment would they give?

  Similarly if the test did not confirm the diagnosis, ask what the significance of a negative result might be.

- Finally, tell them the outcome: *'Mrs Kumar's V/Q scan showed a large defect in the right lung consistent with a pulmonary embolus. Blood tests confirmed a diagnosis of antiphospholipid syndrome. She was treated with low molecular weight heparin and aspirin for the remainder of her pregnancy, and delivered a healthy girl baby at term'.*

(Contd.)

An example of how to plan a case study *(contd.)*

- Give your summary. Pulmonary embolism is an important cause of maternal mortality. The diagnosis can be difficult, and you may have to treat on suspicion. There may be an underlying cause.
- Give direction for further study and open up further discussion (see page 46, Planning to lead a discussion).

  'Some of you may have come across antiphospholipid syndrome. When we next meet we will consider it in more detail, and here is some reading for you to do in preparation. Let's return to the question of…'

FOR THE CREATIVE TEACHER

Run your case study as a debate.

1. Ask four people to prepare different approaches to a difficult case.
2. You chair the debate, introduce the case, and outline the problem. Offer two paths, A and B, to deal with the problem. The audience votes on whether they would follow A or B.
3. Your prepared speakers now talk about these two ways, presenting arguments for each. A1 and B1 start, then A2 and B2 offer further reasons for their preferred way.
4. Allow the audience to ask questions. Then they vote again and see if anyone has changed their mind.
5. Summarize by explaining what you actually did and give the outcome.

Telling the story

Have you ever noticed the effect on an audience when someone recounts a good story? Every one immediately listens. A good story holds its listeners in suspense.

A good story-teller selects only what is essential to keep the story moving, holding back certain bits of information so that you want to keep listening. Think of your favourite crime writer. At the end, you realize the importance of every detail and clue. In fact, sometimes you pit yourself against the author to work out what is going on.

This is precisely what lies behind the presentation of a case as a basis for teaching. Just as all good stories have certain elements that grip the reader—a difficult choice, a dilemma, an apparently insoluble problem—so it is with the story behind a case study.

When you tell a story you need all the skills of good communication that we focus on in Chapter 7: good use of voice, eye contact with the audience, and positive body language. You have to look interested in what you are telling. If you are new to this, practise on your own. Make sure you keep the story of the patient moving. Don't rush it, but don't let it drag. Be concise.

If you are co-presenting a case, you can ask the other person to tell the story. Try not to distract from this by having unnecessary word slides. In fact this is a good moment to use the <B>or <W> key; there is more on this in Chapter 8.

Because you want to focus on one clear message in a case study, it is a good idea to allow time for further discussion at the end, but you need to plan in advance what is relevant to get the discussion going.

Planning to lead the discussion

You may choose to use discussion as part of your teaching. It may grow out of the questions you ask, or you may invite your audience to offer opinions and discuss the salient points as we have suggested during the presentation of a case. A discussion can range over a wide area of the subject, but where it is part of a teaching session you need to guide the discussion so that it stays relevant to your aims. In order to do this you need to set some boundaries for the group and decide how you will keep within them. This requires planning.

In your plan you should think about:

- Where will the discussion go?

  You can use a discussion within the body of any teaching to vary the stimulus. It is particularly useful to fix a controversial point or to wrap up a subsection. More usually, discussion takes place at the end of a presentation, particularly when you have finished presenting a case to peers and seniors who may wish to express opinions and offer other thoughts.

- How much time should I allow for discussion?

  Awareness of time is always necessary. If you are opening up discussion within the case study, you will need to be very strict with time as you need keep moving through the rest of your plan.
  At the end of a session, if you allow more time for discussion, remember that you are responsible for wrapping up the discussion. Repeat your take-home message and close the session.

- What else do I need to think about?

  You must be able to hear what is said, and ensure that everyone can hear too. Repeat the contribution so that everyone can hear it. You must listen to and take in what is being said, and think about how it fits with the main theme. You then choose whether to comment, or ask for someone else to agree, disagree, or offer a further comment, or ask for a different contribution. You should be keeping an eye on the whole group.

- How will I close a discussion and move on?

  Keep an eye on the time. Just before you need to move on warn the group: 'Time for one more contribution'. At the end of that contribution, thank everyone and put up your next slide and move to the front of the group to draw their attention back to you and your next section.

(For difficulties that can arise when leading a discussion see Chapter 11.)

Participation is an essential part of adult learning so use discussion to focus the students' attention and as a way of including all learners. You guide it to encourage a wide range of contributions.

Time to stop and think

- Where will I keep a list of case studies I want to use for teaching?
- When will be a good opportunity to teach using a case study?
- What will be the single most important take-home message from the case?
- How can I become a better story-teller?
- At which points in the presentation will I interrupt my narrative to ask questions?
- Which points will I want to pick up later for discussion?
- How will I be ready to lead the discussion?
- How can I use slides most effectively for a case presentation?

Notes for Trainers

How to prepare case studies for teaching

Always use a case you have been involved with. Never make up a case that did not actually happen.

This training session needs to follow straight on from a well-presented case. Your trainees need some immediate experience of what you are talking about. Liaise with the presenter and make sure you have their outline beforehand.

Aims

- To understand the elements of a case study
- To learn how to construct a case presentation
- To begin to understand how to include interactive elements.

Outline for the session

Time: 30–40 minutes
Resources: slides, hand-outs

1 A real case presentation
2 Trainer input
3 Tasks
Sample slide set.

1 A real case presentation

You must have a case as a model for discussion and analysis.

2 Trainer input

Interactive analysis of the case using the slides. First, identify key elements of structure and, second, make clear the skills needed to present. This may be the first time that your trainees have thought about structure and teaching skills rather than the content of the talk. This will be a major shift in their thinking. As you talk about the skills that the presenter exhibited, point out the times on your course programme when you will be helping them to learn those skills.

3 Tasks

TASK I

This is a task to get your trainees to think about interactions and questions in the middle of a case.

1. Find a moderately suitable written/ published case study from your specialty.
2. Prepare a hand-out by photocopying or retyping the case report.
3. Remove the title and name of author. (For this initial exercise you do not need to produce your own case.)
4. Add the following questions:

- Q1 If you were going to present this case to an audience, what would be your main teaching aim or take home message?
- Q2 At which points might you want to get your students to stop and think about alternative ways of treatment or management? Mark these on the text.
- Q3 What questions could you ask? And where? Write them by the text.
- Q4 What points would you pick up for a further discussion afterwards?
- Q5 What title would you give this case?

Give everyone adequate time to read the case and answer the questions. When most have reached Q4/5, reveal the actual title of the case. Then lead a general discussion to see if there is agreement on Q1–Q4. Ask whether they would want to use that particular case. You should give your personal reasons why you would or would not consider this case suitable.

TASK 2: PREPARE A 2-MINUTE MINI CASE STUDY

Trainees present the outline of a case, which they choose from their own clinical practice.

In their 2 minutes they must state what the case is:

- why they found it interesting
- the main difficulty and what options they considered.

They must also:

- prepare one question to ask the rest of the group
- tell the actual outcome
- produce a summary slide which states what they think is the most important feature of the case, and a useful web site to find out more.

TASK 3: STORYTELLING

Time: preparation 15–20 minutes

3 minutes per story + 2 minutes for feedback

(See notes on giving feedback in Chapter 7, page 93 and Chapter 9, page 112).

This task is about taking one element of a case presentation and giving an opportunity to practise:

- on their own, trainees prepare a story about a real patient, which they personally found especially interesting
- divide them into smaller groups of five or six
- give them 3 minutes in which to set the context and then to describe the case without notes.

NB: The case history becomes a way of gaining or maintaining attention. One purpose of this activity for trainees working in a second language is to build confidence in the use of spoken English.

TASK 4

If your course requires trainees to make a presentation and lead a discussion, find an opportunity for them to stand at the front and lead a short discussion. It could be about some social activity—the content does not matter. What does matter is becoming comfortable in front of a group listening, commenting, and taking contributions.

Here are some slides for trainers to explain what we mean by case study:

What do we mean by case study?

A case study—a vehicle for teaching based on real experience
It offers opportunities for interactions and discussion

What is a case study? A medical mystery

- You reveal clues
- You guide your audience to the right conclusion
- It is memorable

What is in a case study?

Thinking about content
How to choose a suitable case:

- What was interesting for me?
- What did I learn from it?

Other considerations

- Interesting
- Unusual
- Dilemma, problem, crisis
- A decision to be made
- Something to learn

What do you NOT do?

- Do NOT tell everything there is to know on this topic

What are the key elements of a good case study?

- Introduction
- The story of the case
- The moments of decision
- A question on ways of proceeding
- The patient outcome
- The main message
- Further discussion

Thinking about presentation

- Careful planning
- Interactions
- Good-quality slides
- Timing
- Control of questions and discussion

Summary

Why do we use case studies?
The best vehicle for inspiring and effective teaching

CHAPTER 5

How to prepare interactive teaching

In this chapter you will read about a number of ways of moving away from a traditional lecture format. As with every aspect of teaching we have discussed so far, preparation is the key to confident, interactive teaching. You will find ideas for taking small steps towards changing the way you teach, for example by beginning a teaching session with a question. You will also find information on developing good question techniques and material on planning to divide a large group into small groups.

Interactive teaching: what, when, and why

QUESTION 1: WHAT DO WE MEAN BY INTERACTIVE TEACHING?

Any teaching where the teacher and students interact with each other, or where the students interact together, is interactive teaching. In fact, if you are inventive, you can always create interactions in your teaching whatever teaching method you choose. Here are some examples:

- a brainstorm to see what students already know
- questions and answers for revision or consolidation
- discussing options during a case study
- using questions while demonstrating a skill (Chapter 10)
- small group discussions
- a course where the material is already generally known and well organized, for example Advanced Life Support (ALS).

QUESTION 2: IN WHAT SITUATIONS IS INTERACTIVE TEACHING POSSIBLE?

With any size of group

It works best in groups of up to 12; it is very possible in a group of up to 30. Even with an audience of 100, there are ways in which you can interact with one section at a time. You might say, 'Here is a question for the men', or 'Here is a question for the first two rows or back two rows'. You just need to be clear about who should answer the questions.

At any time during your teaching

Questions can be used at the start of a session. This will help you assess what the students already know before you move on to either the main part of your lecture or to a series of teaching questions. For example: you want to know if your students have learned some basic anatomy. Go round the group asking them in turn to name one nerve, bone, or artery.

Interactions can be used half way through a case presentation (onlined in Chapter 4). For example: you present a case history, and then ask: 'What do you think happened next? What tests should be done now?'

At the end you may ask: 'What is important to remember from today?'

In any type of teaching room

There are interactive elements you can use in a large lecture theatre—you can ask students to discuss in pairs.

In a more flexible space, you can divide one large group of 50 into two halves and give one half a task, for example some questions requiring written answers, while you lead a question and answer session with the others. At half time, you swap the groups.

QUESTION 3: WHAT ARE THE ADVANTAGES OF INTERACTIVE TEACHING?

Perspective of the teacher

- to involve your students in the learning process
- to keep them alert and keep them thinking
- to help you judge the level of student knowledge
- to give you feedback on how well you explain things
- and to learn from students—there may be things you had not thought of!

Perspective of the student

- gives them confidence
- trains them to respond rapidly.

QUESTION 4: WHY MIGHT THIS WAY OF TEACHING BE PROBLEMATIC?

Perspective of the teacher

- difficulty of not covering all the material
- less control over the group
- the group may be silent
- demands skills you do not yet have
- loss of authority
- takes longer to prepare.

Perspective of the student

- fear of not knowing
- fear of making a mistake.

SO WHY SHOULD YOU MAKE THE EFFORT TO LEARN THIS SKILL?

If relationships are at the heart of good teaching, interactive teaching fosters these. Good teaching should always be an interaction between the teacher and the learner. Your responsibility as the teacher is to dispel the fears students may have of learning this way.

Think of teaching as fulfilling a number of expectations on both sides. The teacher expects the students to listen, speak, reflect, question, remember, apply, participate, and think critically. The student expects the teacher to teach them well, take their difficulties seriously, learn their names, appreciate their efforts, and get them through exams! Interactive teaching fulfils all these expectations—and more.

Active participation in learning is more interesting and more effective than passive learning.

Interactive teaching: making a start

Once you have sorted out your aims and content, you should always consider how and when you can introduce interactive elements. It is possible across the spectrum of teaching methods from the formal lecture to the clinical demonstration with one individual. The more you teach interactively, the more you should aim to reduce the amount of teacher-talk and increase the level of student participation.

For those new to this style of teaching, here are some ways to introduce an interactive element at the start of a teaching session. They all start with a question.

It is a good idea to have a flip chart or board handy to write up responses. (See Chapters 6, page 73 and 8, page 104 for hints on using this effectively.)

1. **Open brainstorming**
   You ask a question. You receive one answer per student in any order, from as many as possible.
   Brainstorming is not the whole teaching session, it is a way of collecting as many ideas as possible from your students.
2. **The ring doughnut!**
   You ask a question, then you go systematically round the group asking for one point from each student. This is a more controlled way of brainstorming.
3. **A written answer**
   You write up a question and give students a few moments to write an answer. You ask them to raise a hand if they have an answer, and you pick a number of students to give an answer.

4 **A vote**
Ask the group: how many of you would do XYZ? Hands up!

These four simple suggestions for opening teaching with a question require a question with many possible answers. Such questions might be:

What are the causes of ...
What are the differences between adults and children when ...
What are the signs ...
What are you going to consider if a patient presents with ...

FURTHER IDEAS FOR GETTING STARTED INTERACTIVELY

- Students write down answers in pairs. They turn to another pair, and share their information thus adding to their original ideas.
- Students write answers; you ask one student to read an entire list, others tick off similar responses. You ask only for additional ideas. This keeps the session moving and does not take too long.
- Students write answers; you show a list you have written up earlier and students compare their answers. This can be done with very little talking.

WHAT DO YOU DO WHEN YOU RECEIVE THE ANSWERS?

- You respond positively with thanks or a smile. Try not to be judgmental and avoid saying: 'No, that's wrong.' unless the information could lead to dangerous results.
- Avoid saying 'OK' to every response.
- Aim to write down exactly what is said. You may use a scribe to do this. Ask permission to change or shorten wording. Get more explanation if it is unclear. You direct the scribe what to write.
- Welcome ideas you had not thought of.

HOW DO YOU MOVE ON ONCE YOU HAVE THE ANSWERS?

- If you have written down students' answers in a structured and organized way to fit your prepared outline, you can now continue with your more formal lecture using the structure provided by the students. From one initial question you have the core material to develop your topic.
- Realizing students' ignorance, you may need to take a step back and fill in the gaps in their knowledge!
- Write up answers randomly. Once you have collected the key points for the topic, ask the students to discuss in pairs the correct order or a good structure for this knowledge or treatment.

This approach is helpful before written examinations that require short answers or an essay.

WHAT ARE THE STUDENTS DOING?

They are participating, thinking, and speaking.

> When starting a session interactively, be flexible and be open to new ideas.

A conversation

Before we move on to aspects of planning to teach a whole topic through questions and answers, look at the sample dialogue in the box. Notice that the questioning is a form of a conversation between a teacher and an individual or class, in which, by careful choice of questions, the teacher uses the student's existing knowledge, and helps them to organize it in a clear and memorable way.

Example of a conversation

Teacher	We are going to talk about the cardiovascular system in pregnancy.
Student	I don't know anything about that.
Teacher	Let's see; what is the function of blood in general terms?
Student	Well, it carries oxygen and nutrients round the body.
Teacher	Excellent: and in pregnancy how many bodies have to be supplied with oxygen and nutrients?
Student	Two, I suppose, the mother and baby.
Teacher	So what will be needed to do this?
Student	More blood!
Teacher	Exactly. During pregnancy the volume of maternal blood increases by 40–50%. How does the blood actually get to the mother's organs and the placenta (and hence to the baby)?
Student	It's pumped by the heart!
Teacher	So do you think the heart pumps the same quantity of blood per minute in a pregnant woman as in a non-pregnant one?
Student	I should think it has to pump more.
Teacher	You're right!

We could go on, but you see how it works. Notice that almost all the information came from the student, even though he claimed not to know anything about the subject.

Here is the same information presented as a slide.

CVS in pregnancy
↑ oxygen demand
↑ circulating volume 40–50%
↑ CO
↓ SVR

Which method will give the student confidence that they know it?

Interactive teaching: preparing questions

You have decided to teach a group interactively in order to *engage* them actively in the learning process. You want to encourage maximum participation. We have suggested interactive ways of starting a topic, now we come to some tips on preparing questions for teaching a whole session interactively. Before you get to the point of turning your teaching material into questions, take a moment to remind yourself of the six steps of good preparation. It is only once you have chosen clear aims, selected the content, found a simple structure and a clear message that you can start planning the questions to get the message across most effectively.

DIFFERENT TYPES OF QUESTIONS

1 Closed questions

Closed questions have one answer or a simple list of one-word answers. Words that start a closed question are: When? Does ...? Name ...?

Examples:
- What structures lie in the femoral canal?
- What is the incidence of diabetes in the general population?
- When did the spots appear?
- Does she have brothers or sisters?
- How long have you been studying?
- Give me some examples of
- Tell me what you do next
- Describe the characteristics of
- What are the causes of
- When are you going to …?

what is the purpose of closed questions?
- to get facts in order to test or reinforce knowledge
- to build on what people know already
- to build confidence in the students.

2 Open questions

Open questions may be answered in a number of ways. They may have a number of right answers. The response may be a point of view or an opinion.
Question words that start an open question: How? Why? What if?

Examples:

- How would you check …
- How do you decide if …
- Why would you not …
- What is happening to the patient when …
- What assumptions are you making?
- What might happen to the patient if …

what is the purpose of open questions?

- to develop understanding and to stimulate thought
- to learn to apply knowledge and develop problem solving
- to help people make good judgments.

In practice you will often ask a simple closed question and then immediately follow it with a supplementary open question. For example:

- 'If X happens, what else must you think about? Why?'
- 'What is the dose for…? How will you know if you have given too much/too little? What will you do if that happens?'
- 'What would be the treatment of choice? How will you give it? Are there any alternatives?'

You can read more on questioning which offers a hierarchy of thinking if you turn to page 69 where there is a brief outline of what is called Bloom's taxonomy.

Remember to get answers from more than one student so that you hear what as many of them as possible think, and to give every student the opportunity to speak at least once.

HOW TO PREPARE THE QUESTIONS

It is helpful to turn to your textbook, Oxford Handbook, or other source of information. Use the information in this book as the basis for formulating your questions. Turn every statement into a question.

Check that you have a variety of the different types of questions we have outlined above. Start with a simple question and then ask more demanding questions.

If you are following a teaching syllabus, you can involve your students in preparing for an interactive teaching session. Give them the relevant passage in the Oxford Handbook in advance. You prepare your comprehension questions on the passage and prepare to expand the parts that you expect them to find difficult. By teaching in this way the students cover the content twice.

Points to consider are:

Do I write out the questions in advance?

This is a good idea if you are not fully familiar with the material or if you are new to this way of teaching. Check that you move from simple to complex questions and make sure your questions offer an adequate challenge and are not all too simplistic.

Do I wait for the answers?

Yes. Give adequate time for people to respond, try not to answer the question yourself but keeping the session moving, while you keep an eye on the time.

How do I plan a summary for a flexible session?

Because you have planned and know in advance what you want the students to remember, when you come to the end, you can get the summary from the students with a series of questions: Where did we start? What were the key points you need to remember? What difficulties might you encounter? Reinforce this with points already written out on a flip chart or a final slide.

What are good ways of questioning?

- a supportive environment
- clear questions
- pitched at the right level, not too hard, not over simple
- the teacher involves everyone
- the teacher repeats the question and if necessary rephrases the question
- the teacher gives time for the students to answer
- the teacher asks a number of people the same question—either to demonstrate that everyone has the right idea, or to show there are a number of different answers.

What are bad ways of questioning?

- asking 'where shall we begin?'—it makes you look indecisive
- intimidating one student or even the whole group
- having over-long, rambling questions
- making students feel stupid or humiliated, for example by expressing dissatisfaction with an individual's level of knowledge
- making jokes at the expense of one person
- impatience, not waiting for the answer
- not listening to the answer or even acknowledging it.

The way you lead a question and answer teaching session can build or ruin your relationship with your students. If you say something you regret, say sorry immediately!

WHAT ARE POSSIBLE DIFFICULTIES?

Some students never speak

If you know you have a shy or weak student who never speaks, use the doughnut method and take that student's response early on. If you get students to write answers before speaking, look specifically at what that student writes and be encouraging before getting spoken responses.

One trainee knows it all and dominates the group

If you have a know-all in the group, take their response last. If necessary tell them you want to hear from others in the group.

Be confident and take steps to control the group.

You think teaching this way takes too long

Plan the timing and work on the principle that less is more. You might cover less but the students will learn and remember more.

Any time you need to move on, simply take 10–15 minutes to teach some detailed content or explanation as necessary. At least you won't be doing that for an hour.

Ground rules for asking questions

Always plan to keep control of the session by setting out ground rules.

You decide how many answers you will listen to.

Tell the students to listen to each other.

Ask students to raise their hands should they all call out together.

What if someone asks a question you cannot answer?

Do remember to allow students to ask questions! If questions are asked to which you do not know the answer, then you and the students can aim to find out together. The best teachers go on learning.

If you encounter other difficulties when you first try any of these ideas, turn to Chapter 11, page 135 on finding solutions.

USING A FRIENDLY OBSERVER TO GIVE YOU FEEDBACK

It can be helpful to have a friendly observer. This person can make notes on how often you ask questions, and how long you wait for answers. If you give them a seating plan they can mark it each time someone gives an answer. Afterwards you can see at a glance who spoke most and if anyone never answered. You can also see whether you have a tendency to allow the men or women to speak more!

Interactive teaching in small groups

An excellent way of creating interactive learning is to divide a large group of students into small groups of fewer than six.

STUDENTS WORK IN PAIRS

The smallest groups are pairs of students. You can involve a whole lecture theatre full of students in learning together by setting a question at any stage in a formal lecture, telling them to work with one other person, and giving them a specified length of time to discuss the answer.

The key to success is knowing how to regain their attention. One way is to put up the question as a slide on a coloured background. When you want their attention, press the <W> key, and they will stop talking.

You may ask for volunteers to give you answers. Always ask for answers from a number of students so that they become accustomed to speaking out and knowing that there may be a number of acceptable answers. Write any good points on the flip chart.

If you have taught a large amount of factual information in the previous teaching session, and you intend to build on this knowledge, use a warm-up revision question at the start of the next lecture, which the students answer in pairs. This should focus their attention. The quickest way to move on is to show your prepared answer. Their active revision at the beginning, will keep them concentrating.

Paired discussion is an appropriate way of learning during a case presentation. Tell your audience how long you are giving them to answer a question in twos, and what signal you will give for them to stop talking, before you resume your presentation according to your plan. Always keep the time short for these interactions. A maximum of 2 minutes is usually enough.

SMALL GROUPS FOR REVISION

Revision can be done very effectively in small groups if you give different questions to different groups. The reporting back is more interesting if everyone has been given a different question to answer. The answer must be concise, and you may produce some model answers on slides or as a hand-out.

You may choose to offer oral examination practice in small groups. You select some students to be examiners, and ask them to prepare some questions (with a few suggestions). They then lead a question and answer session. You are free to observe and listen. Afterwards reflect on the process as well as on any gaps in knowledge. The more responsibility you give to the students, the better prepared they are for their professional life.

SMALL GROUP TUTORIALS

You invite one student to lead the session with a prepared case study or paper.

WAYS OF USING SMALL GROUPS DURING A FULL DAY MEETING

When you run a meeting you do not want to end up with a day filled with formal lectures. Plan to have sessions in smaller groups at least once during the morning and afternoon. You will need to give group leaders clear instructions, especially about content and timing. You must also plan in advance how you will divide up the participants. You can do this by adding a letter or number to their name badge to indicate the group, or allow them to choose and sign up on arrival. Do limit the number in each group.

Allocate a faculty member to time-keeping and moving groups. This person should try to give group leaders a 2–3 minute warning before the end.

Here are three suggestions:

1. A Faculty member leads a series of discussions. Your group leaders have a number of scenarios prepared in advance. They change the item for discussion every 10–20 minutes according to prior agreement.
2. Groups remain in the same place and Faculty rotate through the groups. Variety comes through the person and the topic. This is effective as fewer people have to move around.
3. Groups rotate. This is the best method if there are a number of demonstrations requiring equipment. You must allow at least 2–3 minutes for groups to move.

When a group leader has to deliver the same material three to four times in succession to different groups, there is a danger that the amount they include will progressively increase due to the inclusion of new points raised by successive groups. It is vital for the leader to have a short written list of key points. In the few moments between groups, the leader must use that time to think, 'If I add this point, which one will I leave out?'

PLANNING THE ROOM

If you have a flexible teaching room and you plan to do interactive teaching in small groups, anticipate how you want to set out the room. Even if you teach in a fixed-seat lecture theatre there are ways in which students can interact with each other for the benefit of their learning.

Time to stop and think

Have a go at this question quiz.

1. What percentage of total teaching time does a typical teacher spend asking questions?
2. What percentage of teacher questions require simple remembering of facts?
3. What is the usual time a teacher waits for an answer to a question?
4. Who is the person most likely to answer the teacher's question?
5. What is the typical ratio of questions asked by the teacher to questions asked by the trainee?
6. What percentage of classroom questions remain unanswered?

(Contd.)

The answers are on page 67. Did you get them right? What surprised you? Which area most reflects the way you use questions?

- What is stopping me from doing more teaching in this way?
- Do I really think the students learn if I take them through a series of questions?
- When am I going to try out one of the brainstorming ideas?
- Which areas of my teaching are most suitable for turning into interactive sessions?
- When am I going to try it out?
- How can I introduce group work into my teaching?
- Who can I ask to observe and give feedback?

Notes for Trainers

How to prepare interactive teaching

As with every area of training, you must illustrate interactive teaching when you present this material. With this in mind, much of your input has been written as a series of questions for you to ask. You must draw the answers out from the trainees. By this stage in your course, you should be able to ask them what examples of interactions they have noticed in the course so far. There is too much material for a one training session. You must select according to the time available. We suggest an outline for a single session. If you have time for two sessions on interactive teaching then follow the two-stage outlines.

Give your trainees an immediate opportunity to teach interactively. Make them put what they have learned into practice.

Aims

- to convince trainees of the benefits of interactive teaching
- to give trainees the tools to teach interactively
- to develop good question techniques
- to allay trainees' fears
- to understand how groups work
- to produce more creative teachers.

Before you start: room and resources

- Change the layout of the room for this session (see Chapter 2, page 23)
- Get flip chart and pens, and/or board, chalk/pens, board wiper
- Prepare flip chart sheets in advance with headings
- Photocopy sample hand-out Appendix 4 Hand-out 2

Outline for a single training session on interactive teaching

Time: 90 minutes
Resources: slides, Oxford Handbook, Hand-out 2, Appendix 4

1. Introduction with trainees giving examples of interactions
2. Trainer input: explain the mechanics of brainstorming, asking and receiving answers
3. The question quiz and thinking about questions
4. Tasks
5. Discussion regarding practicalities and difficulties, and time for reflection.

For a fuller explanation of these steps, please select from the notes on the two-stage training below.

Outline for two sessions

For trainees who have never taught interactively we suggest you take this material in two stages.

STAGE I

Time: 90 minutes
Resources; slides, flip charts, pens, Hand-out 2

1. Introduction
2. Brainstorming—good points and fears
3. Short slide presentation
4. Illustrate two interactive tasks by role-playing actual teaching situations
5. Pause and reflect on what you have done
6. Summary slides
7. Task: a trial brainstorm
8. Final comments and time for reflection

Sample slide set.

STAGE 2

Time: 90 minutes
Resources; slides, flip charts, pens, Oxford Handbook, Hand-out 2

1. Revision
2. Slides: the question quiz, page 67
3. Trainer input with hand-out: thinking about closed and open questions

4 Tasks
5 Practical issues
6 Discussion and time for reflection

Additional material: Bloom's taxonomy.

STAGE I

1 Introduction

5 minutes

Stress the importance of this part of their training; that if they put into practice what they learn about interactive teaching, this will make a big impact on their teaching. This session is designed to get them thinking creatively about fresh ways of teaching.

Ask: what examples of interactions have you seen so far?

By starting with a question and getting the trainees to give you examples, you are in fact demonstrating the open brainstorm method.

2 Brainstorming—good points and fears

5–10 minutes

- Write on to separate flip charts good points and fears concerning interactive teaching.
- Lead this brainstorm by demonstrating the doughnut model.
- Choose a scribe with instructions to note only one word if possible.
- Give the group a moment to think.
- Explain what you will do.
- Go around the class.
- Each trainee gives one answer and you accord each answer equal merit.
- You give them permission to say "pass".

3 Short slide presentation

5 minutes

Ask the students to compare what you thought of beforehand and show your slides with their lists. Tell them you will return to their fears later.

See page 71 at the end of these notes for suggested slides.

4 Illustrate two interactive tasks by role-playing actual teaching situations

Choose appropriate topics from your specialty for introducing a topic by brainstorming.

ROLE-PLAY I

5 minutes

You pretend to be a teacher and actually demonstrate

Sample topic: difficult airways

Introductory question: How do you anticipate that an airway will be difficult? (Equally you could ask for causes of diseases or injuries.)

Use the doughnut method and go around the class receiving as many answers as possible.

Keep this brisk; do not spend too long on it.

ROLE-PLAY 2

5–10 minutes

This role-play demonstrates a different way of using an opening question, a way which will help any trainees who lack confidence.

Introductory question: Think about what is the same and what is different when you prescribe for children rather than adults.

Divide the class into four groups.

Explain very clearly that groups1 and 2 list what is the same, and that groups 3 and 4 each list what is different.

Join groups 1 and 2 who now share their ideas.

Join groups 3 and 4 who share their ideas.

The two larger groups should have prepared a long list.

Ask each group in turn for one response. Keep information coming from alternate groups until their lists are finished.

We have found that groups enter into the competitive spirit of this activity.

This method works well for considering advantages and disadvantages in any topic.

5 Pause and reflect on what you have done

10 minutes

Perspective of the trainee:

How did you feel as trainees working in this way?

What did you like about these two activities?

What did you not like?

Perspective of teacher:

Why was this a good method to choose?

Talk about the methodology.

Talk about the choice of starter question.

- Get them to see what has happened. Look at all the information they have generated which is on the flip charts.
- Talk about what they will do next and how they might organize this material.
- Give advice on the practicalities of receiving feedback and the need for clear writing on boards or flip charts.
- Look back at the list of good points and fears to see if they want to add anything or ask a question.
- If time allows, let them discuss how to meet and eradicate the list of fears.

6 Summary slides

Round this off with your final slide which contained your aims for the session. Then put up a slide with the final task 7.

7 Task: a trial brainstorm

30 minutes

- Give trainees a task to prepare in pairs and allocate time to perform it interactively.
- Select from the Oxford Handbook enough topics for every pair of trainees. Label the topics A, B, C, etc., with a page reference.
- Give a different topic to each pair.
- Each pair works out:

  an opening question to put to the whole group

  a method to do this from the new ideas you have given them.
- Tell them that one person will lead, one will write up answers.
- When the trainees present, keep timing very tight. Only about 1 minute is needed per pair. You will have to interrupt to keep things moving, as every pair has a turn. As you observe, make a note of any point you wish to make when you give the group some feedback.

8 Final comments and time for reflection

You should be able to praise the trainees for having attempted this task successfully. Point out how lively the session has become and that interactive teaching is possible. Review the outline for the session and how it was constructed. Finally point out their success in presenting their question. Give explicit feedback on the importance of:

- planning a good question
- being confident
- looking at the whole group
- giving very clear instructions
- speaking loudly enough
- keeping to time
- legible, clear, and neat writing.

If writing was illegible or poor in a previous task ask your trainees to practise during a break!

Remind them never to give instructions when people are talking.

STAGE 2

1 Revision

Remind the class of the steps to good preparation—ask them what they are! Ask them to remind you of the advantages of interactive teaching and the many different ways of doing it.

2 Slides: the question quiz

Make six question slides (page 71) and allow time for written answers. Make a second set of slides (7–12) and this time the answers should appear.
Discuss what you learn from this and what is surprising.

What percentage of total teaching time does a typical teacher spend asking questions? 3–4%	What percentage of teacher questions require simple remembering of facts? 82%
What is the usual time a teacher waits for an answer to a question? 0.9 seconds	Who is the person most likely to answer the teacher's question? The teacher
What is the typical ratio of questions asked by the teacher to questions asked by the trainee? 50–100 : 1	What percentage of classroom questions remain unanswered? 30%

3 Trainer input with a hand-out: thinking about closed and open questions

- With a colleague illustrate a question and answer teaching dialogue by reading aloud together the conversation on page 55.
- Using the gapped hand-out, which you will find in Appendix 4 page 195, do some work on asking good questions. Explain that almost every statement we make when we teach can be turned into a question. When we plan an interactive teaching session, we begin with our aims, content, structure, and summary, then we see how much of it we can turn into a series of questions.
- Briefly outline good and bad ways of asking questions.

4 Tasks

TASK 1: PRACTISING WRITING QUESTIONS

10–15 + 10 + 10 minutes

- Set a teaching context. Give the same teaching topic from the Oxford Handbook to every trainee.
- Each trainee writes out the key points they want their students to learn. Then they turn each statement into a question. They should end up with five to six open and closed questions.
- Now they work in pairs.
  They ask each other their questions.
  They discuss the questions and pick the best.
- You ask for their best questions and write up a selection of these in order to discuss why they are good questions.
- Remember to reinforce the idea that a closed question can be very useful if followed by an open question.

TASK 2: PREPARING A WHOLE INTERACTIVE TEACHING SESSION

This is suitable if there is time for private study to prepare.
Resource: the trainees should agree a topic that they all teach and refer to the relevant section of their Oxford Handbook.

- Planning an interactive teaching session from scratch.
- Before you look at the textbook:
  What is your main aim? Is your take-home message clear?
  What will be your sub-headings for reaching your goal?
  What might you need to revise?
- With the content in front of you in the Oxford Handbook:
  What will be your brainstorming question at the start?
  How will you organize this?
  How will you develop the questioning to cover the rest of the content?
  Write the questions you will ask.
  What might you need to actually tell them?
  How will you get your students to sum up?
  What further learning resources will you need to prepare or direct them to?
  How will you arrange the room?
  What do you want to write on the board or flip chart?

You may wish to print these instructions for each student.

5 Practical issues

If you have not yet done so, talk to the trainees about practical considerations:

- rearranging the room, the tables, and seating (see Chapter 2 Preparing the room, pages 23–25)
- use of board or flip chart (see Chapter 6 Flip charts, page 73)
- receiving answers
- other problems the trainees raise (see Chapter 11).

6 Discussion and time for reflection

Assessing tasks and giving feedback

Here are some things for you to make notes about during their training tasks in order to give effective general feedback on interactive teaching.

1. What did they do well? Did they have good questions? Did they ask a variety of questions?
2. Have they made progress with eye contact, voice, presence, and confidence?
3. Do they include the whole class when asking questions?
4. How did they start?
5. How did they handle responses?
6. How did they handle extra noise?
7. Was the flip chart used well?
   What about quality of handwriting?
   Choice of colour?
8. What one bit of advice will significantly improve their next bit of teaching?

Additional material

BLOOM'S TAXONOMY: A WAY TO THINK ABOUT LEARNING

Bloom (1956) described a taxonomy or classification of forms and levels of learning. Anderson and Krathwohl (2001) summarized the main ideas: that effective learning starts at the lower level and eventually achieves the higher level. They described three domains of learning: cognitive learning about knowledge, affective learning about values, and psychomotor learning about doing things. Bloom gave most attention to the knowledge domain and least to the affective.

The **knowledge** taxonomy in its current form looks like the diagram in Figure 5.1.

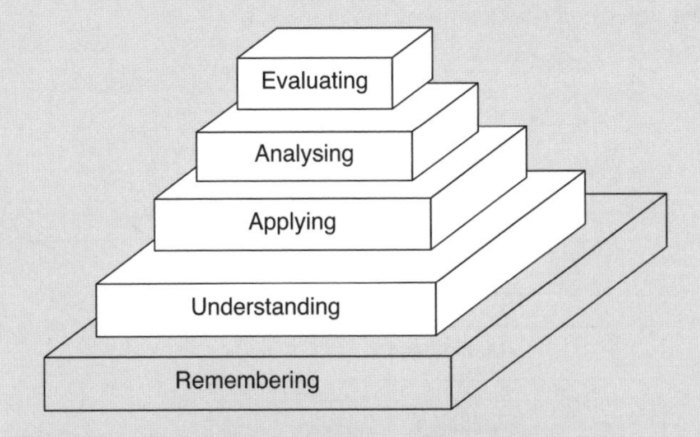

Figure 5.1 Categories in the cognitive domain of Bloom's taxonomy (Anderson and Krathwohl, 2001).

When designing questions as part of our teaching or as an assessment, the taxonomy can be used to look at the level of complexity we are working at. Trainees progress up the hierarchy of knowledge as they progress in their speciality, starting with simple remembering of facts.

It also suggests a way of categorizing levels of learning, in terms of the expected ceiling for a given programme. Thus training for technicians may cover **knowledge**, **comprehension**, and **application**, but not concern itself with analysis and above, whereas full professional training may be expected to include this and **evaluation** as well.

The other two domains are less well known but worth examining.

The **affective** taxonomy, which deals with values, looks like the diagram in Figure 5.2

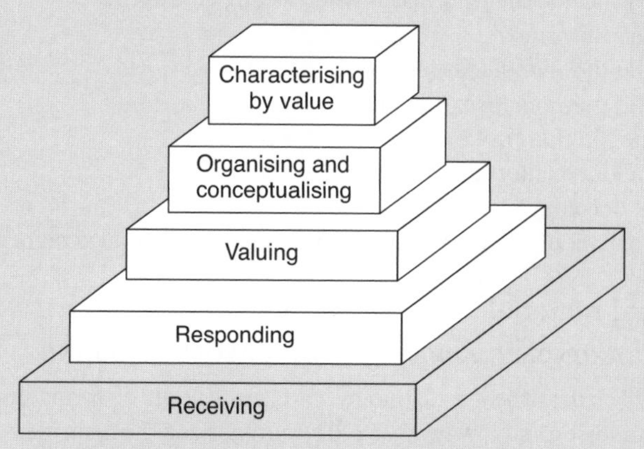

Figure 5.2 The affective taxonomy.

This might seem more difficult to apply but it is part of the knowledge, skills, and attitudes of competence. It is about how we learn our attitudes in our professional life.

Finally the **psychomotor** taxonomy; Bloom never completed this work, but others have suggested the taxonomy in Figure 5.3.

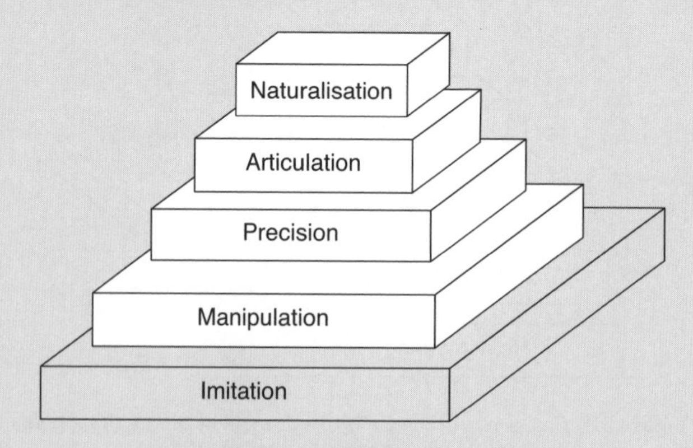

Figure 5.3 The psychomotor taxonomy.

This emphasizes the importance of copying or imitating an expert, through to the point at the top where the skill is 'natural', performed without having to think consciously about the component parts. This is our aim in teaching a clinical skill as described in Chapter 10. The skills have to be broken down into small steps. We have referred elsewhere to the analogy of learning to drive a car. What is a simple process now, was not so when first encountered. This too is the whole purpose of this book: to break down the facets of teaching skills so that you come to teach well without thinking what you are doing all the time.

These classifications are interesting and can be useful, but are not prescriptive. They are useful when thinking about what you want to achieve with your trainees and the way you want your teaching to develop.

Sample slides for Stage 1

These slides would benefit from some additional pictures or cartoons.

Teacher	Student
• most important person • talks all the time	• listens • does not interrupt • does not ask questions • never speaks

What is the difference?

- I am learning
- I am being taught

One is active
One is passive

Why do interactive teaching?

- It involves the learner
- Learner is more likely to remember

What is it?

Can you give examples of interactive teaching on this course so far?

Move to flip chart and look at advantages and disadvantages

Advantages for the teacher

- Check students' knowledge
- Learn from the students
- Build relationships
- Students: engaged in learning
  remain alert
  learn to think
  learn to make decision

Why might we fear it?

- Anxiety
- Less control over group
- Won't get through material
- Demands skills I don't have
- My lack of knowledge might be revealed
- Silence—no response …

When is it best?

- Small groups up to 30
- Type of teaching
  - discussion
  - exam revision
  - consolidation and repetition
- Time of day: end of morning; after lunch

How do I start?

With an open question
A good first question is essential

(Contd.)

Question and then ...

1 Brainstorm
2 Doughnut
3 Small group task
4 Competition
5 Vote
6 Write down and then report
7 Debate

Any other ideas?

Reflection

- How do you feel about it?
- Did you prefer it to having a lecture?
- What did you not like as students?

Can you guess what MY aims were?

- To convince you of the benefit of interactive teaching
- To give you the tools to start.

Have I succeeded?

CHAPTER 6

How to prepare extra resources

Now is the moment to turn your attention to teaching resources, because now you have completed your preparation of the content and decided what teaching method you are going to use. You need to choose what is most appropriate from what is available. If you use a variety of resources and visual aids in creative ways, you will hold the attention of your students and they will enjoy your teaching more. This is an area of teaching in which to be creative and take risks.

Choosing teaching resources and visual aids

WHAT RESOURCES MAY BE AVAILABLE TO YOU?

pen and paper
chalkboards and whiteboards
flip chart
slides.

Although most of us use teaching aids in line with current technology, teaching principles do not depend on technology. We are not including the overhead projector (OHP) as it is rarely used nowadays. It is an example of a technology that has almost disappeared from use. In formal situations all over the world Powerpoint presentations through computer linked projectors have superseded this equipment. It is possible that in the future the same may happen to data projectors and Powerpoint, but the principles of good visuals are unlikely to change.

WHAT VISUAL AIDS MAY BE AVAILABLE TO YOU?

charts
drawings
pictures

items of clinical equipment
models
the patient.

WHAT IS THE PURPOSE OF VISUAL AIDS?

Visual aids are there to aid your teaching; they do not do the teaching for you. They should help your students learn and they should add a dimension that you cannot convey through words.

HOW CAN VISUALS HELP?

- Some students find it easier to remember if they see what they hear.
- Medicine has a specialized vocabulary—students need to see words that are new to them.
- Some things, such as formulae, charts, and essential data, are better shown than described in words; for example the structural formula of steroids or the calibration curve of a blood gas machine.

PRINCIPLES

1. Decide which resources you want to use.
2. Plan how you are going to use these in your teaching.
3. Get everything ready before you start.
4. Do not expect the visual aids to do the teaching for you.
5. After your teaching ask yourself:
   (i) *Was the extra resource necessary?*
   (ii) *What did the students learn from it?*
   (iii) *How can I make it better next time?*

MAKING YOUR CHOICE

Your teaching method will largely determine your choice of resources and the content will determine the sort of visuals you need. Try to avoid the assumption that everything you plan to say must appear on a slide. Formal meetings generally expect slides. We will explain how to prepare these well. They should be used primarily to show data and visuals. If you are teaching interactively and want to write up responses, then you need something to write on. A board is always less wasteful of paper. The big advantage of the flip chart is that you can write things up beforehand and they are ready for you. Presentations of case studies will probably require more than one resource. When you use different resources you vary the stimulus. Switching from a slide to a large clearly printed chart is one way of doing this.

Visual Aids in Clinical Teaching

Most of our teaching time is in a clinical setting. Have you ever used a visual aid in a clinical teaching session?

Drawing

Most clinical teaching is done in small groups, so all you need is a sheet of paper and a pencil. Getting the students themselves to draw is another way of making your teaching session more interactive. Drawing is also a good activity to help students learn anatomical details, since it obliges them to look at the subject in a detailed and systematic way.

HOW CAN YOU INCLUDE DRAWINGS WHILE YOU ARE TEACHING?

If you were to teach airway skills, you could practise drawing the series of four pictures in Figure 6.1, overleaf. You do the drawings, while explaining aloud what they represent.

For a larger group it may be more convenient to use a whiteboard or flip chart. To help you draw quickly and clearly there are two things you can do in advance:

1. Have a small-scale draft of the drawing to refer to when making the flip chart drawing.
2. Make a faint pencil outline on the flip chart of the key parts of your picture in advance.

A good visual approach to chest trauma is to use a flip chart.

1. Draw an outline of the thorax (Figure 6.2, overleaf).
2. Brainstorm with the audience:
   'I've drawn an outline of the chest wall. What structures of the chest wall can get injured ?' (ribs, vessels, sternum, spine, diaphragm)
   'What is the mode of injury?' (sharp, blunt, crush, deceleration)
   'What are the pathophysiological effects of those injuries?' (pneumothorax, pain, respiratory failure)
   'How would we treat them ?'
3. Extend your drawing:
   'Now what about the contents of the chest cavity?'

Repeat the questions: *'What structures can get injured? What is the mode of injury? What are the effects of those injuries?' As the students mention them, draw the structures.*

The second illustration shows how your picture might evolve when discussing a patient with fractured ribs, who develops a tension pneumothorax with pulmonary collapse, mediastinal shift, and tracheal displacement.

Pictures

Why are pictures attractive? What sorts of thing do students learn best from a picture?

A picture should clearly show what you want, and ideally nothing more.

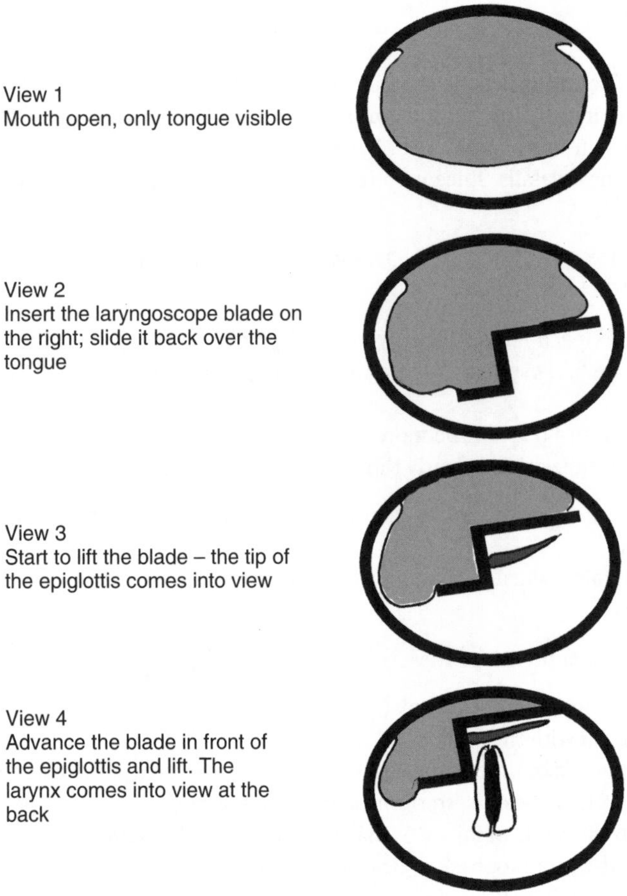

View 1
Mouth open, only tongue visible

View 2
Insert the laryngoscope blade on the right; slide it back over the tongue

View 3
Start to lift the blade – the tip of the epiglottis comes into view

View 4
Advance the blade in front of the epiglottis and lift. The larynx comes into view at the back

Figure 6.1 Teaching laryngoscopy with a simple drawing.

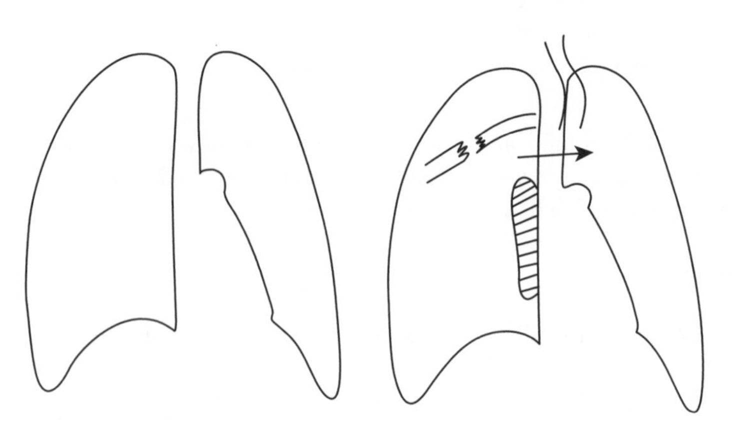

Figure 6.2 Visuals for teaching chest trauma.

Two pictures of a carburettor are shown in Figure 6.3. The photograph contains too much detail, as well as other elements that are confusing and irrelevant. The diagram, in contrast, shows only what is essential, and needs little or no further explanation.

(a)

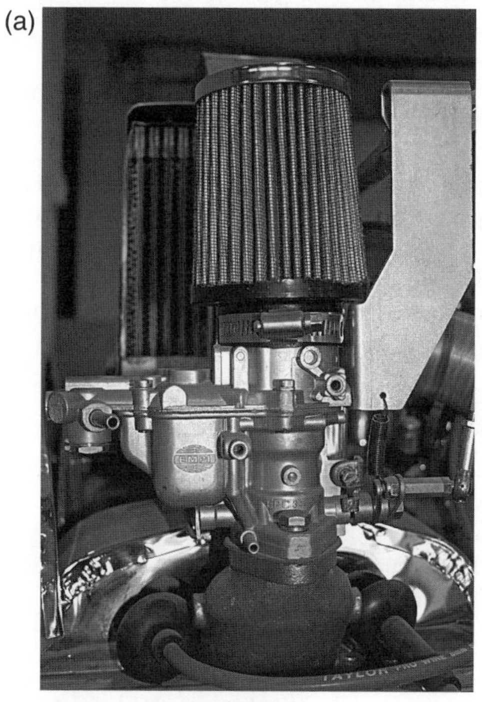

(b)

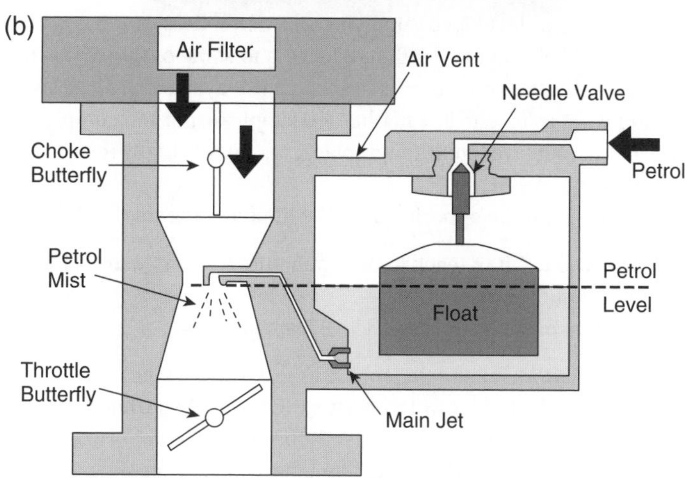

Figure 6.3 (a) A photograph of a carburettor. (b) A drawing of a carburettor.

SOURCES OF PICTURES

You can make your own, get them from colleagues, copy from books and journals with a photocopier or scanner, or get them from the web. What are the advantages and disadvantages of these sources?

For planned clinical teaching sessions why not have a folder in which you keep useful visuals, photos, diagrams, and hand-outs.

Clinical equipment

If you are teaching a clinical procedure that requires equipment, for example intravenous cannulation, plan in advance how to integrate the equipment into your teaching. Be aware that as soon as you show a piece of equipment, the students will focus on it and not listen to what you are saying!

What do you want the students to learn specifically from seeing the IV cannula? This could include:

- opening the pack in a sterile way
- the way you hold the cannula
- range of sizes, and what you might use them for
- the technique of entering the vein
- how to secure the cannula.

Always focus on those aspects the student is likely to find hardest—in this case probably the insertion and manipulation of the needle and cannula.

Models

A whole industry has developed supplying plastic replicas of parts of the body for training, and it is likely that you will have access to some of these. It is important to think carefully about the benefits of using one, if it is available. Is it designed to show the things you want to teach? Is it neither too simplistic nor too complex? Think how you will use it—models are attention-grabbers, and may actually result in the students giving less attention to you.

Look at Figure 6.4 on the opposite page, the lumbar vertebrae.

- How would you use it to teach lumbar puncture to a first year resident?
- What are its limitations?
- How could you make it a focus of active learning?

Most models only work for one student at a time. If you pass the model round the class, the student who has the model will stop listening to you. You could leave some time at the end for students to examine the model. Notice also that important bits of anatomy are missing from the model of the spine—spinous ligaments, meninges—and recognize that you will have to teach about these structures as well. The model is not enough.

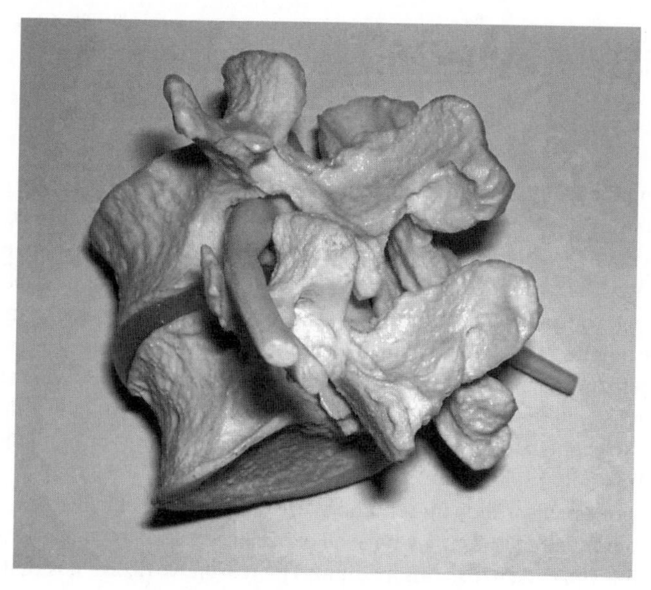

Figure 6.4 A model of the lumbar spine.

IMPROVISED MODELS

Here are some innovative models.

- You can demonstrate the anatomy of the larynx using your hands as a model.
- Some people use a banana to simulate passing a needle through the ligamentum flavum. This is because everybody has a mental picture of what the inside of a banana is like.
- A raw potato demonstrates that a bevelled needle never passes straight ahead, but always deviates to one side.
- A folded sheet of paper can be used to demonstrate the anatomy of the inguinal ligament.

Patients

Patients are plentiful, realistic, inexpensive to use, and often not only willing but positively helpful. For success you will need:

- Consent—so you must explain what you propose to do, and who the students are.
- Cooperation—explain to the patient that you and they together are going to help the students learn something. The patient is not a passive model but an active teacher. The key relationship is between doctor and patient, the subordinate one between teacher and students.
- Gentleness—explain to the patient that you will not be doing anything painful. If they need to undress, tell them how much will be revealed.

When possible use a pointer rather than your hand to demonstrate anatomy.

Use a marker where appropriate to draw on the patient's skin. This makes it much easier for the students to visualize structures underneath the skin.

Slides

We are using the word slides to mean any image you project. In most cases this means using a data projector and Powerpoint or similar presentation software. Do not think you always have to use slides. There is a place for these. They can be prepared quickly once you know the structure of your teaching. You may use them for just one section of your teaching, so think very carefully about whether they are necessary and whether they will be helpful. If you are speaking to a group whose own language is not the same as yours, then putting up words is very important. Students may miss what you say, but if they see it as well they have a second chance to understand. You must then stick to your script, so that what they read reinforces what they hear. (For more on language issues see Appendix 1, page 183.)

Let us be honest, most slide presentations are boring and ineffective. We should not need to be reminded of this, as we have all experienced it many times, yet we and all our colleagues continue to use this medium. The reason we dislike it is that when just words appear on the screen we either read the written words, or listen to the speaker, and as one medium distracts from the other, our concentration weakens. By the end of the presentation we are not sure what we remember.

Why is this so?

- The slides seem to be giving the talk.
- Every slide looks the same.
- Every point is given equal emphasis.
- Information overload: too many slides presented too quickly.
- The teacher cannot see the audience because it is dark.
- The teacher tends to face the screen, instead of looking at the students.
- The success of the presentation depends on the function of an unfamiliar and untested machine.

We all need to change. This involves changing:

- the way we prepare
- the way we present (see Chapter 8).

Nobody is so bad that they cannot improve their technique, nor is anyone so good that they cannot improve their technique.

Beware! There is a danger that when you have learned these lessons you will become overcritical of all future slide presentations. Remember that once you have learned how to prepare and present well, your responsibility is to demonstrate the skill you have learned and teach it to others.

Preparing good slides

Good preparation can change slides from a curse to a blessing.

The slides are not the talk, so do not start your preparation with a blank computer screen and a blank brain. If you do, the computer will take over and your slides and talk will be the same as everyone else's. Start with pen and paper. Follow the six steps to good planning outlined on pages 26–30.

Now decide which parts of your presentation need visual aids. Find the pictures that you need. If you make them yourself they may not be beautiful, but you have 100% control over the content. For those parts of the presentation that do not need visual aids, you need to focus your attention on your interactions and awareness of when to vary the stimulus; you need to focus the thinking of the students on the ideas and message of your teaching.

In general you should not have slides on the screen for more than 50% of your talk. You do not need a slide on screen when you are introducing yourself and the subject, teaching interactively, and taking questions.

The slides are not your notes. If you use them as notes:

- You will have too many text slides—boring.
- The students will know what you are going to say before you say it—even more boring!

Slide design: dos and don'ts

Do:

- Keep things simple. You are a professional clinician, not a graphic designer.
- Choose a slide design and template that is simple.
- Use plenty of diagrams, graphs, charts—you're making a *visual* aid!
- Choose a colour scheme for text slides with a good contrast between text and background, e.g. yellow or white on blue, white on black.
- Stick to four to six lines per slide.
- Use animation only rarely, for example to bring up one line at a time on a text slide.
- Save your final version as a Powerpoint show (pps). Don't start your presentation in 'edit' view.

Do not:

- Use noisy animations. Such things are a distraction for the students and they do not like them.
- Use more than two fonts per slide. The simple rule is to use a sans serif font, e.g. Arial, for headings and a serif font , e.g. Times, for body text.
- Use all capitals.
- Use more than six words on any line.
- Allow elements on your slide to distract attention from the point you are trying to make. The slide is there to help the students, not to draw attention to its wacky colour scheme, flashing lights, over-animations, or dramatic transitions.

Never:

- Use red for text as it is the hardest colour to see on screen.
- Underline—emphasize sparingly, using italics or bold.

Occasionally you may want to put a longer piece of text on the screen, such as a quotation. If you do so, you must pause and allow time for the audience to read it, or read it aloud yourself.

YOU MUST HAVE A PAPER BACKUP

Assume that the projector will fail. In addition to emergency use, a paper backup does two things for you that a screen cannot do:

1. It gives you a map of where you are. Suppose your slide printout occupies four pages for a 20-minute talk, but 10 minutes into your talk you notice you are still on page one! This gives you early warning that you are running slow, and enables you to choose which topics and slides to leave out. (Going faster will not work, you will lose the audience if you rush.)
2. It allows you to move directly to another section of your talk, or to select a supplementary slide, for example in response to a question.

TIMING

Experienced lecturers using slides nearly always find that the actual presentation takes 20% more time than when they practised it. So if your allotted time is 30 minutes, the talk should not last longer than 24 minutes when you practise.

You will then be worried that you will not have enough to say! Think about it—have you ever heard a lecturer criticized for finishing early? Have you ever even been in a lecture that finished early?

USING PICTURES ON SLIDES

The best thing about Powerpoint is its ability to show pictures.

As a general rule, at least a third of your slides should be pictures or diagrams. Pictures are interesting, but make sure that in the pictures there are no major distractions.

If all your slides contain only words, you probably should not be using slides at all—instead write the words on a hand-out that the students can annotate while you talk. (See Chapter 3, page 31 on ways of preparing and using hand-outs.)

Photographs can take huge amounts of computer memory, and may be slow to load; you need to learn how to use photo editing software to reduce file size. No photo that goes into a Powerpoint presentation needs to be bigger than 500 KB (resolution of 72–96 dpi).

If you copy pictures off a web page be very careful because web images are often of very low quality. They may only work if the computer used for your presentation has Quicktime installed and in our experience most do not. Don't copy an image directly from the web into Powerpoint. Save it as a jpeg file on your hard disk, then import it into Powerpoint using Insert > Picture > From File.

HERE IS SOMETHING YOU CAN DO NOW

Find a set of text teaching slides and review them. Do you need to modify them? Could you:

- replace some of the 'words-only' slides with pictures
- cut the amount of text on each slide
- cut the number of slides; if you have more than 20 slides for a half-hour talk, identify what you can cut completely
- vary the stimulus by switching from slides to a flip chart
- identify two slides out of the final five that you could 'drop' if time is short?

If you feel we have been overly critical of Powerpoint, we suggest you Google 'Powerpoint weaknesses' and read the first page of over 400,000 hits! See also www.lifeafterpowerpoint.com

Flip charts

There are huge advantages to using a flip chart rather than slides:

- no technology to go wrong
- less preparation time.

However do not think there is no preparation to do. It is always worth stopping to consider how best to use a flip chart before you do so.

Here are some advantages of the flip chart over a fixed board.

- Writing or diagrams can be prepared in advance.
- The stand can be moved around, so the students see more easily.
- You can tear off a sheet to keep what has been written on it.

However, if you want to write a lot, then the paper is used up fast because the surface area is small.

If you are teaching interactively then you will probably choose to write on a flip chart. Do remember that you can use a flip chart to make something clear at any stage of any lecture with slides. It is a way of varying the stimulus. Plan how you will write on it so that the end result is clear and helps students to remember and understand. Avoid letting it end up a complete mess.

Please do not write in capitals. Doctors often do this because their normal handwriting is unreadable. Capitals are slow to write and difficult to read. Take time to practise neat lower-case printing. (For more on the use of flip charts see Chapter 8.)

Always make sure there is enough paper before you start.

Always move the stand to a position where everyone can see it. In most seminar rooms you can only use the top of the paper as the lower part is not high enough to be read.

Buy your personal set of clearly named flip chart pens and always keep them with you.

Boards

Chalkboards or whiteboards

The big advantage of boards is that they are reusable. If you know you are going to use a board, plan how to make the best use of it—otherwise you will cover it with a jumble of words and pictures, which will not help anyone.

Usually, you will use it for technical terms, for a rapid diagram, data, or an equation. As with the flip chart, you can write on it to clarify or expand a point at any time during a slide presentation.

There is no point writing anything if the students cannot read it.

- Write large enough for all to see.
- Write neatly.
- Do not write in capitals.
- Use black if possible on whiteboards, occasionally blue; only use red for underlining or bullet points. Red is invisible to those sitting at the back of the room.
- It is very difficult to write neatly on a shiny whiteboard, so do practise.

WHAT DO YOU NEED?

Never assume there will be pens or chalk in place—even less a board wiper!

- Carry your own chalk or set of pens around with you.
- Have more black pens than other colours.
- Make sure you buy and use only *dry wipe* pens.
- Keep hospital alcohol gel or nail varnish remover handy—if you pick up and use a permanent or flip chart marker by mistake, this will remove it.
- Bring your own board wiper—a damp paper towel from the nearest washroom.
- Clean the board when you finish ready for the next person.

> If your writing is bad, you need to practise.
> Always remember to bring your own materials.

Interactive whiteboards

Your department may have invested in an interactive whiteboard (IWB). These are common in school classrooms throughout the UK. An IWB combines the best uses of slide projection with the advantages of a flip chart, all linked to a computer. If you have one, it can be a helpful tool for interactive teaching. You can 'interact' with the board and appear to write or draw on the screen.

Before you use it in front of students, find the instructions and work out how to use it: how to show slides; how to bring up the next slide; how to write on the screen; and how to clear the screen. Make sure you know where the 'pen' is to be found. You must always use this special writer. Never use a normal felt pen with ink in it.

WAYS OF USING IWBS

- You can show slides you prepared in advance in the normal way. If you have a question that you want the students to answer, you can write up responses with the 'pen'. Of course you have to know how to clear the board before the next slide.
- Any work you write up can be saved on your computer to be used another day or turned into a hand-out. This is especially helpful if you want to build on the work done previously. If you are brainstorming and want to keep the results, what you have written can be saved as a Word document on your computer.
- Resources for boards can be excellent if you choose software with a library of pictures or images.
- You can show video clips, pictures, and prepared slides, just like any screen.
- It is helpful for small interactive sessions as students can write, type, or drag things around on the screen.

Time to stop and think

- Do my regular resources actually help my teaching and my students' learning?
- Can I produce simple drawings for a clinical procedure that I teach regularly?
- What do I most need to change regarding my slides?
  - the layout
  - the content.
- How can I vary the resources I use?
- Do I need to improve my writing? When can I practise?
- Which one thing can I do to be more creative?

Notes for Trainers

How to prepare extra resources

This is an enjoyable, interactive, and practical session during which you will observe enormous progress in your trainees. The session moves from simple to complex visual aids, from drawing on a piece of paper to slide preparation and presentation.

Keep stressing the principle that visual aids are there to help, but not to do the teaching for you. You have to demolish all the bad practices that your trainees have seen and absorbed over the years, while still helping them to respect their teachers. Above all, you must show excellent slides, while demonstrating that they are not necessary for the whole teaching time. We suggest that you talk about visual aids in clinical teaching without any slides. You need to prepare a set of clear slides to reinforce the dos and don'ts of slide design.

Before this session, tell your trainees they will need their laptops and ask if they would charge the battery before the session, as it is unlikely that there will be enough sockets.

There is some overlap with Chapter 8, which focuses on using the resources. You will probably combine the material so read Chapter 8 before you start.

Aims

- To encourage students to consider how resources and visual aids help in all teaching methods
- To give opportunities to practise creating good visual aids
- To improve slide design and preparation.

Outline for the session

Time: 2–2 ½ hours

Resources: individual laptops with slide sets, flip chart paper, felt pens, possible hand-out

1. Introduction to resources and visual aids
2. Trainer input on visual aids in clinical teaching
3. Tasks: drawing
4. Trainer input on preparing good slides
5. Task on improving own slides
6. Time for discussion and reflection

Hand-out: text from http://www.lifeafterpowerpoint.com. This was previously on the BBC website.

1 Introduction to resources and visual aids

Start interactively by asking the trainees to come up with the resources and visual aids listed at the start of this chapter. Find out what they use most and what is new to them. Draw out the role of visual aids, using the early part of the chapter. Ask why they should be using them. Try to distinguish between the resources, i.e. the equipment, and the actual visual, i.e. the picture, chart, or diagram.

2 Trainer input on visual aids in clinical teaching

Using visual aids in clinical teaching may be a new idea. Start with some interactive, question-based teaching. Ask them to describe a visual aid that has helped them. They will certainly not mention a text-only slide. Make a mental note of this and remind the class of it when you do get to talking about slides! Give them the ideas on different types of drawings, equipment, and the patient. If time allows, ask them to copy your simplest drawings.

3 Tasks: drawing

TASK 1: DRAWING

- Give the students a topic, for example induction of anaesthesia. Ask them in pairs to list the pictures and diagrams that would be helpful in teaching the subject. These may include:
  graph of anaesthetic gas uptake
  equations
  diagrams and pictures of machine, breathing circuit.
- Now get them to list the sources they would use:
  own photos and drawings
  colleagues materials
  books and journals
  internet.

TASK 2: DRAWING ON A FLIP CHART

- Divide the students into groups of three or four.
- Set the context.

Example 1: you are going to teach nurses to suture a scalp wound.

- Prepare visuals to demonstrate:
  wound preparation
  local anaesthesia
  suture insertion
  knot tying.

Example 2: you are going to teach trainee surgeons the insertion of a gastroscope

- Prepare visuals to demonstrate:
  the positioning of the patient
  the anatomy of the oropharynx and upper oesophagus
  structure and controls of the instruments
  some sample views in both diagram and photographic form.
- One member of the group will present the drawings as if actually teaching.

Points to make when giving feedback:

- What is good about the drawing?
  good labelling
  good use of paper
  good use of colour
  legibility of handwriting.
- What do the drawings actually show?
- Have they numbered a series of drawings?

When you sum up, before moving on to talk about slides, stress that the trainees can do something they thought they could not do—they can draw—and remind them of the ways to make diagrams easier, e.g. by marking the paper in advance.

4 Trainer input on preparing good slides

Point out to the class *'We are x minutes into our teaching session, and I haven't used a single slide yet'*.

Tell them that everybody thinks they are a creative genius when it comes to slides but they need to focus on the basic principle that slides are there to help people learn. You have to put over a negative message, that much Powerpoint teaching is hopeless, in a non-threatening way. Then you must demonstrate very positively that by changing a few simple things, they can make a huge improvement. They need to understand that they themselves must become good models for the future, and that people who have poor technique have simply not been shown how to do it better.

5 Task on improving own slides

- Get the trainees to find some slides of their own. They can take any three or more slides and work on them for 20 minutes, aiming to make them simple and clear. This is an opportunity for you to go around and listen to them as they now critique previously used slides.
- Encourage them to experiment with different backgrounds and to get the opinions of others.
- When they have completed the changes, ask them to load the original and the improved slides onto the main computer for the final part of the training. (Take precautions against viruses spreading.)
- As many students as possible show their slides. Students may explain what changes they made and why. They may not need to speak—the contrasting slides will speak for themselves.
- Feedback: after each presentation, just the trainer will give any appropriate, short public feedback.

6 Time for discussion and reflection

Now is a good time to distribute the hand-out for everyone to read before they leave. After an active session, it is a good idea to have a few minutes of quiet reading time. Have a discussion about any difficulties they foresee when they put changes into practice. Ask them to make notes on what they have learned in the whole session. Encourage them to plan a specific opportunity when they will use a flip chart or board instead of slides; when they will use a variety of visual aids which are not slides; and the three things they want to change in slide preparation before their next presentation.

Summary of Part 2: preparation and planning

A PLANNING CHECKLIST

The talk:

- *Am I clear about what is important?*
- *Is my opening clear?*
- *Have I remembered I need to introduce myself?*
- *Have I made the topic relevant to this group?*
- *Are my points in the best order to achieve my aim?*
- *How will I end?*
- *Does my timing seem right? Have I noted approximate times on my plan?*
- *What can I omit if time goes?*
- *Am I planning to take questions?*
- *Do I need prepared questions to get a discussion going?*
- *Have I suitable visuals?*
- *Do I need to prepare a hand-out?*

What to take:

- *Have I printed out my notes or slides?*
- *Have I a plan for the use of a board?*
- *What else do I need to take, e.g. board writers, memory stick, hand-outs, name badges, Blu Tack®*

Arrival:

- *What is the teaching room like?*
- *What do I still need to do when I get there?*

TEACHING PLANS

We are all different. We approach the question of teaching notes differently. Some people like very detailed notes and write out their plan. There is no shame in having teaching notes. They have the advantage of saving you hours of preparation the next time you teach the topic. After you teach you can make immediate changes for next time. Other people are happy to work from headings, either because they know their material so well or because they are able to think very quickly on their feet. There is no single right way.

It is traditional in some parts of the world to learn a talk by heart. This is demanding and time-consuming. Far better to have written at least your main headings, listing smaller points you do not want to forget. Do write out your opening sentence, in case your mind goes blank as you stand up to speak.

If you are showing slides, you must have a printout of your slides. You can mark onto these your approximate timings, additional points, reminders about when you want to switch to a flip chart.

Part 3

During your teaching

Introduction

Now that you are ready to present your fully prepared session, you must do it justice when you teach. Before we turn to good delivery skills, we want to remind you again that you will always find something that is less than perfect when you teach, which you can improve next time.

When you teach, you have to reckon that you are in the entertainment business. Like good entertainers, you have to get and keep the attention of the audience. We have looked at ways of doing this through content and teaching method, now we turn to skills you can learn and improve that help you maintain attention during your teaching.

To get your message across effectively, you must make use of the personal skill set you were born with. These are sometimes called communication or presentational skills. In Chapter 7 we give you tips about good body language, and ways of using your voice and eyes to get your message across more memorably. As you learn how to put these top tips into practice, your teaching will improve immediately. You want your students to concentrate on what you teach, not on your peculiarities. In Chapters 8 and 9 we return to resources and how to use them. We introduce thinking on the use of simulators as an educational tool. Chapter 10 takes a different area of teaching, teaching a clinical skill. We end this third part with some solutions for difficulties you may encounter, especially when you begin teaching interactively.

You can never be quite sure how you come across when you teach and there are a number of ways of finding out. We touched briefly on feedback in Part 2. However, we introduce the topic of feedback in more detail in Chapter 7 as it is so important and is an integral way of improving your teaching. You can begin the feedback or reflection process by asking yourself a couple of questions immediately after you teach, or by asking a friend to give you feedback on these questions:

- What did I do well?
- What do I want to change?

If you are really keen, you might like to ask a friend to make a simple video-recording.

Part 4 of this book will look in greater detail at the many ways we can evaluate teaching and learning and why we learn from feedback.

CHAPTER 7

Getting the message across

Teaching is not about 'the force of my personality' or 'being born a teacher'. There are skills relating to your posture or stance, your eyes, and your voice that you can learn, control, and change. As you read about them, note why they are so important to getting your message across. These skills are fundamental to the way you communicate your teaching to your students.

If you are working through the book on your own, rather than on an education course, concentrate on just one of these three areas each time you teach.

Stance—what you do with your body!

When you face your students, you need to present yourself as confident and relaxed. Stand comfortably, with your feet slightly apart. If you are nervous, breathe deeply two to three times before you start. Then smile. When you smile, you relax. You need to give the impression of wanting to be there.

Do:
- stand tall
- stand still
- stand where everyone can see you and where you can see everyone
- smile, relax, and enjoy yourself!

Do not:
- use distracting mannerisms
- hop from one foot to the other or cross your ankles
- stand in front of the screen or flip chart.

Never:
- stand with your arms folded in front of you
- stand with both hands in your pockets; it looks sloppy.

SITTING OR STANDING?

Only sit if you have a small group and you want to teach quietly and informally. When you sit down, you change the atmosphere in the room.

Standing enables you to project your voice more easily. It is more formal. It is always better to begin teaching a new group in a more formal manner, and then move to greater informality. When you are standing, you can move around more easily. You may need to move to the board or to a different position in the room if one group cannot easily see you.

PRACTISE

Look at yourself in front of a mirror and practise standing comfortably:

- feet slightly apart for balance
- shoulders back
- back stretched tall.

WHY IS BODY LANGUAGE IMPORTANT?

- Confidence: if you *look* confident, you will *become* confident.
- If you are confident, your students will have confidence in what you teach.

FEEDBACK

If a friend is observing ask them to comment on whether gestures were helpful. They can also note any repeated mannerisms, for example waving your arms around or pacing up and down like a polar bear in a zoo.

Eyes—how and why you maintain eye contact

Learn to look consciously at all sections of the class. When you keep your eyes on your students you have instant feedback on how your teaching is going. It is a real joy to have their full attention and to interact through eye contact.

Do:
  look up
  look at the group
  look at the whole group.
Do not:
  look down to read from notes
  look up and stare at one person
  look out of the window or at one fixed spot on the ceiling
  look constantly and repeatedly up and down.
Never:
  lose eye contact by turning your back to your students.

This means you must never speak while looking at the big screen behind you nor while writing on the flip chart or the board. Therefore never use a laser pointer for text slides—it will only make you turn your back. (See Chapter 8 on Presenting with slides, page 104, for more on this topic). To keep your eyes looking forward at the class, keep your feet pointing at your class. How you place your feet has the effect of making you face the students.

WHY IS EYE CONTACT IMPORTANT?

- Relationships: you cannot build a relationship with your students if you do not look at them. As you get used to looking at them, and as your students feel included, you will get a better response from them. They will be more ready to listen to what you are teaching.
- Responsibility: you are responsible for teaching the whole class, not the wall, nor just a couple of individuals! If you do not notice that your students are no longer giving you their full attention, you will not realize that it is time to vary the stimulus. Noticing what is going on in front of you and responding to it makes you a better teacher.

FEEDBACK

It is particularly helpful to ask a friend to comment on eye contact with the students. He or she will be able to tell you if you focus too much on one group or one spot of the room or if you never look at one particular group. We all have a classroom blind spot. There is one section of the class we do not easily look at. This might be the front or back row, the left- or right-hand side. Once you have identified your blind spot you can remove it! An observer will also pick up if your eyes never stop moving and never look at anyone.

Voice—using your voice to maximum effect

Just as your eyes are directed to the whole class, your voice is always directed to the back row. There is no point teaching if nobody can hear you. You use your voice as a means of gaining and maintaining attention.

- You must get into the habit of projecting your voice (not shouting) and speaking more loudly than you think you need to. You are competing against interior noise from projectors, air conditioning, heating, and bodies soaking up sound, and against external sounds of people talking, traffic, rain, or thunderstorms. Address the back row rather than the nearest row. *Ask* the students if they can hear you.
- Speak more slowly than normal and enunciate more clearly. This helps people to hear. It is even more important to do this, if you and your students do not share the same language. If you know your normal talking speed is very fast, you must make every effort to slow down. (See Appendix 1, page 183 on Using another language.)
- Try to make your voice interesting even though you may find this difficult. You can speak more loudly, more softly, more quickly, more slowly. To underline a point, repeat it more loudly and more slowly. If you are telling a story, rather than giving facts, vary the pace. Should you choose to add an aside, please do not lower your voice. It is very annoying to the back rows if they can not hear what the others are laughing at.

- Use your voice to indicate a question. This is particularly important in a question and answer session led by a non-native English speaker. Make clear by your intonation that you are asking a question, and wait for an answer.

Do:

speak loudly
speak clearly
vary your voice.

Do not:

mumble or speak at normal conversation level
talk very quickly
start loudly and then get quieter and quieter.

Never:

talk with your back to your students.

SOME TRICKS:

- If you are nervous and have a dry mouth, sip cold water before speaking.
- To regain attention after discussions, clap your hands—do not raise your voice.
- Stop speaking if you want to allow students to read any text. Give your students a break from your voice.

WHEN YOU USE A MICROPHONE

Speak loudly, slowly, and clearly. The operator can turn you down, but not up. Your mouth should be about 30 cm from the microphone.

Here is another reason why you must not turn your back on the audience. If you are speaking into a microphone and you turn away from the audience, they will not be able to hear you and the sound of your voice disappears. As you turn backwards and forwards your voice will come and go.

WHY IS VOICE IMPORTANT?

- Confidence: if you sound confident, you will become confident.
- Responsibility: you are responsible for the class being able to hear you.

FEEDBACK

If a friend is observing, they will be able to pick up on verbal mannerisms, for example saying 'Right!' before every instruction, 'Okay' to every student response, 'um' and 'er' constantly, or scattering your speech with the current habit of saying 'like' or 'you know' in every sentence. Your voice is the means of getting your message across. It is a tool to be used to help maintain attention; therefore project your voice. This friend should sit at the back and wave a hand to indicate if you are speaking too quietly and cannot be heard clearly.

The moment when you start

You may have to decide to:

- break in to conversations

- introduce yourself
- ask people to turn off their mobile phones.

This is the moment when you combine all you have learned so far. Stand comfortably. Take a deep breath. Look confident and smile. Your resources are ready. Your opening sentence is written out and placed in front of you. You look around the room. Unfortunately your students are not ready! They are chatting, still arriving, and generally ignoring you. What do you do to get attention?

You attract attention, clap your hands, close the door, move to a different position. You begin to speak, and pause …

Yes you stop for a second and you look around. You continue to look at any group that is still talking, once you have everyone's attention, glance around the room, smile, and begin.

The art of the pause is the art of gaining full attention right at the start.

Now you can begin properly by being clear about what they are going to learn in the next hour or so, and why it is important, and by using what you have planned to make the subject relevant.

Giving instructions

When you give instructions for a small group discussion, you need to put into practice all the above tips and more. Do not speak if you do not have the attention of the whole group. One easy mistake to make when you divide a large group into smaller groups is to indicate groups first and then start explaining the task. This is fatal. Everyone is busy moving, talking, saying goodbye to their neighbour. Always explain the task clearly before you divide people into groups. Have a routine for giving instructions:

1. Ask them to listen carefully while you explain. Raise your voice slightly and speak more slowly while you explain what you want them to do.
2. Tell them how much time they will have.
3. Show instructions that you wrote earlier on a slide or flip chart and give a moment to read and think about the task.
4. Ask if everyone understands.
5. Only now divide them into groups.

You need to stay in control and look confident whenever you do something different.

> Put these ideas into practice and you will improve your teaching immediately. Keep improving these techniques and you will transform your teaching. Your confidence and enthusiasm will be infectious.

Time to stop and think

- Do I stand comfortably?
- Do I feel and look confident?
- Am I aware of the whole group?
- Do I look at them enough?
- Is my voice clear and interesting?
- Do I talk too fast?
- Am I too quiet?
- What am I going to improve first?
- Who will I ask to observe and help me?

Notes for Trainers

Getting the message across

Introduction

This session is very practical and fully interactive. It demonstrates the cycle of learning. Students have observed you teaching; they work in small groups; you give them some direction and reasons for following your tips, they then immediately put into practice what they have discussed and heard in groups of no more than six. You finish the session with time to reflect on what they have learned and what they want to change. Then they set personal targets, which they will aim to meet during the rest of the practical sessions on the course.

It is essential that you have been demonstrating the good practice that you commend.

You need to decide the location of the groups in advance. If the room is large enough, use the main room. Never put only two groups in one room. They will be distracted and listen to the other group. Make sure that the observers are seated looking outwards at the wall from the centre of the room at the person speaking, and that the person on their feet is looking into the room. This means the group concentrates on the speaker from their group only.

You also need a person in each group trained in giving feedback. It is essential that the trainer who leads the group sticks rigidly to time. They must also focus only on the two feedback questions; what went well and what one thing should they change. The trainer will need to keep coming back to focus on the positive as others will want to make negative comments. The reason why it is so important to focus on the positive is that you do not want your trainees to stop doing the things they are already doing well. Praise what is good. This may be counter-cultural but it is an essential part of getting people to change. After listing all the positive aspects, see if the trainee can come up with one thing to change. Remember that after five or six have practised, there will be five or six different things to change as the trainees learn from each other.

There is an outline on giving feedback in these notes under *Additional material*.

Aims

- To develop those communication skills that make the biggest impact on teaching
- To improve the way trainees stand, use their eyes, and their voice
- To give trainees the tools to develop self-evaluation skills so that they know how to go on improving.

Outline for the session

Time: 1 hour +

Resources: flip chart; spaces for a number of small groups; a trainer present in each group

1. Small group discussion
2. Trainer gathers ideas and gives fuller input
3. Slide summary
4. Task
5. Reflection

Additional material: Giving feedback.

1 Small group discussion

5–10 minutes

Begin by asking the whole group what are the teaching tools they were born with. Set the scene by getting them to remember some very bad teaching. Now in small groups, they list what advice they would give relating to body language, voice, and eyes in the form of dos and don'ts which would lead to very much improved teaching.

2 Trainer gathers ideas and gives fuller input

10 minutes

Write up ideas neatly in lists on the flip chart or board. As you do this, discuss and explain *why* this is so important. Add anything that has not been mentioned. At this point do not refer to what we have written on feedback.

3 Slide summary

3–5 minutes

Show a prepared summary on slides. Give your trainees adequate time to read this. Only speak to add points not raised so far, e.g. use of a microphone.

The trainees have now met the material on improving communication skills in three different ways: they have discussed in groups; they have repeated it when they fed back their ideas and you wrote them up; and they have read the text on your slides.

4 Task

30–40 minutes

Allow 5 minutes per person per group

Groups of five or six trainees

- Explain the feedback process and the task before you divide trainees into groups.
- Explain that everyone is going to put into practice what they have learned.
- They will talk on a given topic for 2 minutes only. Give the trainees something easy to speak about, e.g. how they get to work, their hospital, home town, or family.
- After 2 minutes you will stop them.
- There will be 3 minutes for discussion.
- A trainer will be the group leader and allocates a time keeper.
- After 2 minutes the speaker sits down and then answers two questions.

QUESTION 1: WHAT WENT WELL?

It is essential that:

- You explain why this question must be fully explored. You want to reinforce the good points. You do not want people to change what they are already doing well.
- The trainee must try to answer the question first.
- The group leader asks the others to add only further positive points.

QUESTION 2: WHAT ONE CHANGE WOULD LEAD TO THE MOST IMPROVEMENT?

It is essential that the trainer:

- asks the trainee first
- makes a suggestion
- asks the trainee, then the others, if they agree or not
- moves on to the next person.

An alternative method allows everyone to speak one after the other and then the trainer draws out points more generally when everyone has had a turn. If this way of training is very new and radical it may feel less threatening giving feedback in this way. However, it is more difficult to pin point precisely what someone did at the end. If individuals are to make the most of this session, they need to remember the specific feedback that relates to them. We recommend leading feedback immediately each trainee finishes speaking.

The trainer needs to have some experience of observation and feedback. There is more on this below and in Chapter 12.

5 Reflection

5 minutes

Bring all the groups back together.

Encourage everyone to write down

- What they have learned about themselves
- What they most need to change next time they are teaching
- What they learned from watching others.

Additional material: giving feedback

> The observer always starts with the positive, however difficult they find that.
> Limit the number of targets to two at the very most.

Aims:

- To train the trainees to have a conversation with themselves
- To learn how to give good feedback in a positive manner.

This is how you should model this approach:

1. You have agreed the area of observation: eyes, voice, body language.
2. Take notes listing good and bad things and think about only one key area to make the biggest difference to teaching. You must also control the timing very strictly.
3. As the observer, you ask only what went well and encourage the 'teacher' to become self-analytical. Only then do you ask for further positive aspects from others.
4. Ask the 'teacher' what they think is the one thing to improve. If you agree say so and leave it there. If you disagree and there is something glaringly obvious, for example they never stood still, only now ask them where they stood, did they move? Try to get the person observed to come up with the right answer for themselves. The next time they 'perform' in a small group they should have corrected this and you can give them a different target.
5. Move on to the next person. You must control the time for the discussion so that it is the same for everyone.

Sample slide set

This slide set may need some simple animation to bring up some points one at a time. The final slide is one you may or may not choose to include according to time and interest of the group.

Tips For Presenting

Using your body

- Relax and smile!
- Be comfortable
- Look confident
- Make sure they can see you

Do not

- Pace the room
- Develop distracting mannerisms
- Stand where you cannot be seen

Using your eyes

- Look at your students
- Look at *all* your students

Do not

- Turn and look at the screen
- Look only at your notes
- Stare at one person

Beware of your blind spot!

Using your voice

- Be clear
- Project your voice—be loud enough
- Vary your voice—louder, softer, faster, slower

How will you make best use of a microphone in a meeting?

Three questions

- What did I do well?
- What do I want to do differently?
- What have I learned from others?

Additional material: take control of the room!

(Decide whether you want to include this now.)

- Can you be seen?
- Can your slides be seen?
- Can your flip chart be seen and read?
- Is the class seated where you want?
- Is the room a pleasant environment?

CHAPTER 8

Reinforcing the message: using extra resources

Presenting with Slides

This chapter tells you how to ensure that you get the most value from your slides whenever you use them.

As a teacher, you are responsible for controlling the whole environment. That means that you should know how to function in your teaching room; operate the room lights; be aware of how effective the blackout is; and operate the projector and computer that you actually have to use.

Arrive well before you teach in order to check your presentation on the actual computer and projector you will be using—there may be software incompatibilities between it and the one on which you prepared the slides.

Do not be tempted to try and use your own laptop—the time spent fiddling around connecting it up is always longer than you planned. If you leave this until the last moment and attempt to do it just before you start, the audience will get bored and frustrated.

Checking the room

You will already have checked the room as part of your preparation. If you are using visuals other than slides, make sure that everybody can see the screen, board, or flip chart. Move chairs or get the students to sit in different chairs if necessary, but do not start until you are happy that everyone can see. Check how to switch on the computer and projector, and how the lights are controlled. If necessary, ask someone else in advance to do things you cannot reach from where you are teaching.

Note that you need a better blackout for picture slides than for line diagrams or text slides. If the picture is not bright enough, either zoom the projector (to make the picture smaller) or reduce the physical distance between projector and screen.

Where you stand will depend on the room. In a large lecture room you will probably be tied to the lectern because of the need to use a fixed microphone. In a smaller room you may be able to stand more centrally but make sure you do not block the view of your slides.

Take time to adjust your laptop so that it is in front of you and you can see it while still facing the audience.

SOME KEYBOARD TIPS

Save your presentations as a Powerpoint show (pps) file. As soon as you click on the icon, your first slide will come up. If you use a title slide with your name, it should have a white background so that the audience can see YOU as well as the title. Alternatively, as soon as the first slide comes up, hit the <W> key to get their attention while you do your introduction.

There are a number of controls in Powerpoint that will help you. These are available in slideshow view only, either from the keyboard or by right-clicking the mouse. They include the controls listed in Table 8.1.

The <W> or <B> keys are a very powerful way of reminding the students that they have come to learn from you, not to look at your slides. When there is a slide on the screen, they will all look at the screen. When you black- or white-out the screen they will look at you, their focus of attention shifts, and they become more alert! Whether you choose to use a black screen or a white one depends on the room. If the blackout is poor, a black screen is probably best; if the blackout is good, a black screen will plunge the whole room into darkness—you may not be able to find the computer again, so use <W> to provide background lighting.

Keyboards vary, so take time to check in slideshow view what else may be available. On some machines there is a key that takes you straight to the first slide, another that goes straight to the last slide, and two more keys that black the screen out. If your keyboard is non-English the <B> and <W> key functions will probably be different, for example in French they would be <N> (noir) and <B> (blanc). Explore your machine!

Do not overdo this function or it will become irritating. Used occasionally, it remains effective.

> Learn the full range of the keyboard and mouse options in slideshow mode.

Top tips!

1 You know that you have to avoid turning to check the screen to read what is on it. How can you stop yourself? Wherever you stand, *keep your feet pointing towards*

Table 8.1 Navigating within your slide presentation

Next slide	Left-click or Right-click and select or Right arrow or Down arrow or spacebar
Previous slide	Up arrow or right-click and select or left arrow
Slide off / white screen	Press <W> key or right-click and select
Slide off / black screen	Press <B> key or right-click and select

the audience at all times. This will keep you from committing that terrible crime of turning your back on the audience. If you want to keep the attention of the students, you have to make eye contact, and you cannot do that if you are facing the screen. If your feet always point to the students, even if you turn your body momentarily towards the screen, you will automatically tend to turn back.

2 When you show a picture you need to give students time to take it in. Pause for a moment before you start talking about it. This helps them to re-focus on what you are saying, because they have taken in the picture.

Mistakes to avoid

USING A LASER POINTER

This useless gimmick should be banned. It does your presentation nothing but harm. It causes you to turn away from the students. It shows the audience how much your hands are shaking. The tiny red dot is hard for the audience to see. The only time you might need a laser is to direct attention to some detail in a photograph or diagram. After you have pointed to a feature in the diagram, put the laser pointer down. This way you cannot be tempted to commit another crime!

Never start pointing to words as you read. What happens? You turn your back again. This is intensely annoying, indeed insulting for the audience, who can read perfectly well by themselves.

If you need to emphasize something on a text slide, do it by using bold or italic (never underline).

If you need to draw attention to something in a picture:

- put an arrow on the slide
- point with your hand

- use a pointer.

These all work better than a laser because they actually draw the student's eye to the point of importance.

POOR TIMING

This usually happens if you waffle at the beginning, and do not move at a steady pace through the slides. When you then run out of time you find there is no time left to summarize or reflect and you fail to finish strongly.

Noting the time on your printout will enable you to pace the presentation. If you show your summary slide at the time you have noted then you will finish well (see Chapter 6 How to prepare extra resources).

FLICKING THROUGH SLIDES

Do not flick through slides at high speed because time is short, looking for a suitable place to continue. Use the computer controls to go directly to the slide you want. You have planned in advance which slides you will omit if time is short.

What to do when the equipment fails

Remember, *you are in charge, not the machine*. The best approach is determined by how much time you have. The minimum loss of time for a technical failure is 5 minutes.

1. If you have a 10–15 minute slot, abandon the slides and do your talk without. This is the reason why you have teaching notes and a copy of the slides. Do not try and fix the projector, and even if someone else fixes it after you have resumed, do not go back to the slides—you no longer have time!
2. If you have more than 20 minutes ask the organizers to fix the projector while you decide how to shorten your talk. If there is no one to fix the projector go to option (1).
3. If someone is available to fix the projector, give the students a small-group task to do, or send them out of the room for a 5-minute break. They will come back refreshed instead of sitting there becoming impatient.

If you want to read more about this, a helpful website is www.lifeafterpowerpoint.com.

Using flip charts

As we said before there is no technology to go wrong when you use a flip chart. We assume you have come prepared with your pens and that there is an adequate supply of paper.

Take a moment to move the flip chart to a position where the majority can see it.

If you have chosen someone to act as your scribe, make sure in advance that they can write clearly and spell correctly. Whenever possible indicate to them in advance how you want things written up. Having a scribe frees you to move towards the students.

If you are organizing a mass of responses, this is the time to use colour and to number points. Numbering points is helpful and creates order.

If you are planning a series of small drawings, number these. This makes it easier to refer to them.

If you are doing the writing, be aware that you have to turn from the students as you write. If you are right-handed and are alternately writing and asking questions, the flip chart should be on the right-hand side of the room as you face it. Do make a conscious effort to maintain eye contact with the section of the class that sees your back the most. The reverse is true if you are left-handed.

Do not let your writing become too small. Better to keep using fresh paper than to produce a mess that nobody can read.

Colour makes a difference:

- use black or blue for writing
- use red to circle, underline, or number
- use green only if you must
- alternate black and blue if you receive a long list of student contributions.

FURTHER TIPS

- It can be difficult to draw a straight line under a heading; do a wiggly line in red. This also applies to boards.
- If you need to present a drawing, mark it out in pencil before you start—no one will ever see your guide lines.
- You can also note points you must not forget on a page of the flip chart in pencil—only you can see them.

Using interactive whiteboards

Simple things are often the most effective. Some teachers get bogged down trying to do something amazing, when actually simple visuals would engage the students more effectively.

If you are using an interactive whiteboard for the first time, get someone to show you what to do. You must learn how to move forward one slide or go back one. The next generation of British students will all be familiar with this technology from school. They will know how it works!

Using visual aids

Having decided that a visual aid is necessary, the only question that matters is: *can everyone see it?* This sounds very obvious but there is no point in having a piece of equipment or a model if students cannot see. You may well need to get them out of their seats and gather round in order to show them something in detail. Now take a moment to check and ask if everyone can see. This is a way to vary the stimulus. When you send them back they will be ready to concentrate again.

The only reason to use a visual aid is if it actually aids the learning process.

Time to stop and think

- Did I use the extra resources well?
- Do I need to practise with the control keys?
- Did the visual aids make the difficult bit easier to understand?
- Were the visual aids necessary? Did they help to get the message across?
- How can I make the visuals better next time?
- What else do I need to try out or improve?

Notes for Trainers

Reinforcing the message—using extra resources

You may choose to run a whole afternoon on preparing resources, visual aids, and designing good slides. If you do that, have a break between production of improved slides and their presentation. After the break give the tips on presenting, which you will find in this chapter. After hearing these, the trainees can think about how they stand while they present their changes to content. If you return to this topic on a second occasion, we include a good revision exercise, which is more of a competition than a task.

Aims

- To enable trainees to use different sorts of visuals in an effective way
- To help them give good presentations with Powerpoint.

Outline for the session

Time: 40–60 minutes

Resources: data projection, flip chart, pens, two separate rooms, and two laptops

1. Trainer input on presentation skills
2. Tasks
3. Reflection.

1 Trainer input on presentation skills

This part calls for a didactic approach with lots of emphasis from the trainer. The trainees need you to tell them how to do it. Most of them will not know the B and W keys, so put a slide of your own up and demonstrate how they work, as well as the right-click menu in slideshow, and opening a pps file. As the trainer, you must be able to demonstrate effortlessly to the class all the tricks in Table 8.1.

Emphasize the same principles as with all teaching:

- Think about the audience
- Prepare properly—material and room
- Learn how to use the really useful presentation tricks—the B and W keys, to change the pace and focus on the teacher.

Focus on common faults.

Talking about laser pointers can open up discussion.

2 Tasks

TASK 1: SHOWING IMPROVED SLIDES

When each student comes out to speak, you must check that they are looking at the small screen in front of them while talking, not looking behind them. You also need to find ways of correcting them without humiliation, if they turn round to the screen. This is why we make a fuss about pointing your feet at the audience—you can point out quite lightly that the trainee's feet are pointing the wrong way, and they probably won't feel upset.

They should speak clearly and fulfil whatever instructions you have given as regards a commentary, for example you might ask them only to tell everyone the one major change they made.

TASK 2: A WORKSHOP FOR STUDENTS WHO KNOW THE BASICS OF GOOD SLIDES

If you want to revise and consolidate all the good work on improving slides, or if you have a well-informed group, here is a suitable task.

Time: 30–40 minutes for preparation +20 minutes for two presentations and discussion

- Divide the trainees into single-sex groups of seven or eight. (By having men and women working separately there is a greater sense of competition and it is a way of dividing not yet used.)
- Each group works together to produce a teaching set of slides that will demonstrate to others how to produce and present good slides. In other words they are planning to pass on what they have learnt about slide design and slide presentations.

This task demands:

- collaborative team work
- clear thinking and planning
- good time management
- selection of quick-working person on the laptop
- the best person to present.

You will be looking for:

- simple, clear slides
- in a sensible font of adequate size on a well-chosen background

Some helpful guidelines on presentation:

- an introductory and a summary slide with a clear take-home message
- a presenter who looks at the audience and who delivers the slides with pace.

Have fun!

3 Reflection

Give the trainees time to note down what they have learned and what they will put into practice next time they teach with slides.

This is a good moment to remind them that they must not be too critical of other people's slides. They need to show others in future that it is possible get your teaching message across more effectively with a variety of visuals and even without text slides.

Here is an unforgettable take-home message from one group:

'Remember, you are more important than your slides'

CHAPTER 9

Simulators

Hearing the word simulator can produce strong reactions in otherwise calm clinicians—even more so when they hear the word simulator associated with the airline industry. Many extravagant claims are made for simulators. In this chapter we have set out some basic background for those starting to find out about simulators. Perhaps you are deciding whether to go on a simulator course. Perhaps you have money available and want to know if it should be spent on a simulator. We will not give unequivocal answers but try to set out some of the facts.

What do we mean by simulation and simulators?

Simulators and simulation are not the same thing. Simulation is a broad term and it means using your imagination and different levels of equipment to simulate or recreate a situation with a patient.

There are varying degrees of fidelity.

- **Low level** or part skill is using a simple model or manikin to teach a simple skill, for example inserting a urinary catheter. The focus is on learning how to perform a skill or technique.
  There is simple screen-based simulation requiring only software and a computer screen. The patient's pathophysiology is simulated by the computer software.
- **Midlevel** simulation enables the learner to respond with a more complex model in a given context, for example with a resuscitation manikin that can simulate an ECG waveform and measure the effectiveness of CPR.
  Task trainers or part task trainers provide opportunities to learn basic technical, procedural, or psychomotor skills. Procedures such as suturing, intubation, and lumbar puncture can be practised using devices that mimic body parts or regions (e.g. the arms, pelvis, torso) and represent part of a body or system. Once the basic skill has been learned these body parts may then be attached to a manikin to increase the fidelity and enable the student to practise patient interaction during the process.

- **The highest level** or immersive situation is in a simulator. Here you find very expensive equipment, full monitoring devices with live output, in fact everything that you would find in a real clinical situation: a simulated patient, and other staff acting out the roles of surgeon, nurses, or anaesthetists.
  There are student observers, who may be in a sound-proofed observation room, and there is a group of senior teaching faculty, who will give feedback.

Full-body simulation manikins are used to teach cognitive skills and have computer-driven physiological features, for example heart rate and blood pressure. They are able to respond to physical interventions such as chest compression, to drug administration, and drug interactions. The manikin can have either script-controlled physiology within a simulation or the physiology may be automated via computer software.

Virtual reality (VR) simulators are used to improve psychomotor skills in complex procedures that are too dangerous to practise on live patients and give feedback, especially when people have to act as part of a team.

Features of a moderate to high-fidelity human simulator

General features:
- complete human body
- capable of verbal responses
- complete integrated physiological model
- appropriate anatomical landmarks.

Physiological features:
- lungs capable of spontaneous, assisted, or mechanical ventilation
- consumption of O_2, exhalation of CO_2, and uptake of anaesthetic gases
- tongue swelling, pharyngeal swelling
- open/close mouth, trismus
- realistic airway
- respiratory chest wall movements
- synchronized breath sounds
- bowel sounds
- pulses palpable
- heart sounds
- blood pressure measurable
- variety of physiological outputs to standard monitors
- pulse oximetry.

Procedural features:
- defibrillation
- pneumothorax decompression
- cardioversion
- cricothyroidotomy
- external pacing
- pericardiocentesis

- venepuncture
- chest drain insertion
- cannulation
- intramuscular injection
- urinary catheterization
- injection of drugs and responses.

What are simulators used for?

Simulators are generally used in the UK for training purposes—for medical students and junior staff. They provide opportunities for beginners to learn clinical techniques without exposing real patients to risk, and also simulate clinical situations which occur infrequently, for example status asthmaticus, severe sepsis, anaphylaxis, and airway obstruction. They are generally found in university teaching hospitals.

There are two main reasons why simulators are used in the UK:

- It is becoming less acceptable to practise on patients.
- The length of time for training has been reduced, but trainees still need teaching and time to practise so simulation provides an alternative way to learn.

Once a department has invested in a simulator and a team of trained staff, it will usually offer further courses to a wider audience. These courses offer advanced training for teams who work in crisis situations. Crises are clinical events that occur rarely, but are 'high stakes' situations associated with significant morbidity and mortality. Doctors have the opportunity to practise or learn new techniques in a simulated environment.

What can be learned through working in a simulator?

Both technical and non-technical skills can be learned.

Technical skills appropriate to the simulator include procedures such as defibrillation, basic and advanced airway skills, and fibre-optic intubation.

Non-technical skills include team work, exposure to a high pressure, multifaceted environment, and how we deal with it, good communication, interaction with other staff, decision-making, and situational awareness.

WHICH SPECIALTIES FIND SIMULATORS MOST HELPFUL?

Simulators have been found to help teaching in anaesthesia, obstetrics and gynaecology, paediatrics, emergency medicine, critical care, resuscitation, and surgery.

Most initial teaching of laparoscopic surgery is by part-simulation. The first simulations required the student to peel an orange inside a shoebox!

Do the benefits to training outweigh the costs?

The initial outlay for a new high-fidelity 'doll' will be in the region of £250,000 (€295,000; US$380,000). It is worth researching the latest model and its limitations.

It is possible to buy second-hand dolls for less. Then there is the cost of a suitable, dedicated, secure room. The installation costs with wiring, microphones, etc. are in the region of £15,000 (€18,000; US$23,000). However, by far the highest and on-going costs are the staff—the senior teaching faculty of 10 to 12 to run regular courses, and two full-time, permanent technicians. Without technical support you cannot run courses. Each teaching session requires an operator, a nurse, two doctors, and one assistant.

Staffing and location are the priorities and come before purchasing the equipment. Before spending any money, it is essential to gather a team, to get training for everyone in planning scenarios, and experience in giving feedback. Equipment purchase comes after all this.

It is important to think about what courses you intend to run and the specific needs of each of those courses. Do not forget the business plan including when and how you will recoup costs.

High-fidelity medical VR systems can easily cost 10 times as much as lower-fidelity systems and do not necessarily provide superior training benefits. Several less-expensive, lower-fidelity systems may be purchased for the price of a single high-fidelity system, thereby making it possible to train greater numbers simultaneously. Post-purchase support and upkeep are important in learning to control and maintain the manikin and software, and to deal with teething problems.

Whether the results are worth this investment depends on the country. The need in the UK is to find an alternative to learning with patients as training times have been reduced. In a country where it is acceptable to practise on large numbers of patients, then there is not the same need.

HOW OFTEN IS THE SIMULATOR IN USE?

In Oxford, at the Oxford Simulation Centre, the simulator is in use every day, twice a day. It was not always like this—for the first 2 years is was rarely used. It has only been in constant use since the appointment of a permanent operator.

The simulator team

Because of the high cost, your simulator needs to be running full time to be cost effective. In order to do this you will need a large team, some full time, some part time.

THE OPERATORS

Two full-time technician operators are needed to set up, control, and maintain the manikin and equipment during the simulation, do the paperwork, and make bookings.

THE TEACHING FACULTY

It is important to develop credible and competent faculty members who are well trained to use the simulation system and are trained and able to give good feedback. As these people will be full-time, senior doctors you must have a team of at least 10. They will need to fulfil a variety of roles. There is a section on how to observe and give feedback in Chapter 12 page 153.

THE LEAD INSTRUCTOR

The instructor's role is to plan, practise, and run the scenario. A scenario or a debrief can go in any direction and so flexibility and good techniques to redirect the student are key to achieving your aims. Before starting the simulation, this person must brief all those participating.

The instructor must avoid departing from the scripted scenario. This can lead to a loss of direction in the scenario, a loss of confidence on the part of the trainee, and a failure to meet the agreed learning objectives.

THE 'ACTORS'

The nurse and senior doctors involved in the simulator or at the end of a phone must be fully briefed and be familiar with the outline of the scenario.

THE TRAINEES

Anxiety about performing in front of peers and being filmed is the largest hurdle for trainees participating in simulation-based training exercises. Here are some typical behaviours:

- Cavalier attitude, '...because it's only a plastic manikin'.
- Hypervigilance, '...I'm in the simulator waiting for the earthquake to happen'.

Both are totally normal given the situation, but need to be thought about. One typical response from a medical student was that he found entering the simulator the most terrifying moment of his life but that on the reflection the experience was the best bit of his training.

Running a session with the simulator

WHO BENEFITS MOST FROM TRAINING IN A SIMULATOR?

Medical students probably gain most from training with the simulator. They come in groups of about six. Each one takes a turn in the simulator while others observe.

HOW LONG DO THEY NEED?

A reasonable length of time is about 20 minutes. If students come in groups of five to seven, then about 15 minutes for each student in the simulator followed by immediate feedback for 10 minutes is plenty for a morning or afternoon session.

HOW MANY DO I NEED TO RUN THE SESSION?

In addition to the group of students, the absolute minimum number of faculty is two plus one operator.

HOW DO I PLAN AND STRUCTURE A TRAINING SESSION?

- **Who is the audience—medical students or junior trainees?** This sets the level of complexity of the scenario. If it is a teamwork simulation with theatre teams and medical emergency or cardiac arrest teams, it will be highly complex.

- **What is the aim?** What do I want them to learn in the simulator? What do I want to achieve by the end of the feedback?
  Simple, practical aims are best, e.g. how do they explain the procedure to the patient. The learning outcomes must be adapted to the level of the trainees, e.g. if the focus is primarily on non-technical skills and the trainees are experienced clinicians rather than medical students.
- **Which scenario?** You do not have to write every scenario from scratch. It is possible to take a scenario that has been planned and published.
- **What else?** Practise—you yourself must practise the scenario in the simulation centre before any students are present to make sure that it works.
- **Paper plan**. Have a complete lay-out of all possible choices and consequences on paper. This will include:
  - all the information and relevant data for the case
  - a list of each expected student action
  - for each action, a planned reaction.

  At different stages after different student actions, you have decisions to make about the direction of the case, e.g. during a simulation of status asthmaticus you expect students' actions regarding:
  - assessment for severity
  - checking oxygen
  - bronchodilators
  - IV fluids.

  If the student does not check the oxygen, there will be a reaction—the heart rate goes down. If they now respond correctly, you return to the main plan.

The simulation should be fun, and although it is vital that the scenario reflects real life it should not become ridiculous.

The feedback

WHAT HAPPENS AT THE END OF THE TIME IN THE SIMULATOR?

Feedback! Feedback is at the heart of simulation. A good experience of learning in the simulator depends on the quality of the feedback. The goal of the feedback is to help them learn and become better doctors. The specific aim for the session must be kept in view when giving feedback.

It is important to give immediate feedback and to allow adequate time. With the student's permission, the session will be recorded. You can show extracts from the recording to demonstrate points more forcibly, or you can allow the student to watch the whole recording later.

WHAT MIGHT THE STUDENT BE JUDGED ON?

Areas of knowledge:

- gathers appropriate information
- reaches diagnosis, considers differential

- institutes appropriate treatment
- orders interventions appropriately.

Areas of behaviour or response:

- gathers all available information
- anticipates and plans
- calls for help appropriately
- re-evaluates situation
- utilizes team resources effectively
- prioritizes
- concise, directed instructions, closes communication loop
- communicates problem clearly to the team, listens to the team
- manages conflict.

It is debatable how far each area can be given a score. As we have said earlier, better to have a simple learning goal and focus the feedback on that.

HOW IS EVIDENCE GATHERED?

You can only give good feedback if you have the evidence. Three feedback sources can be used in combination:

- the trained facilitator
- the simulation device (e.g. a manikin), especially in procedural simulations
- video recordings.

You will find more on learning through feedback from video recording in Chapter 12.

TYPES OF QUESTIONS

You want the feedback to be supportive, but the student is there to learn. The following questions relate to feedback with an individual.

Some unthreatening starter questions to which you immediately add a further question:
'What did you do well? What else?'
'Did you clearly understand the brief? At what point did you find it unclear?'
'What caused you frustration or discomfort?

Questions that pin-point critical moments:
'Was that a good decision at that point? Why do you think that?'
'Was that action expected?' How could you have responded differently?'
'What was happening at the time? Why do you think they did that?'
'Why did you say or do that? Can you explain your thoughts at the time?'
'What lead you to make that decision? What were you trying to achieve?'

Questions to focus on what has been learned in relation to the aim:
'How could that be improved?'
'What do you think can be improved if you were in this situation again?'

Question to reinforce the take-home message for the individual:

'What is the one thing you need to remember?'

'Are you in agreement with our observations on how you handled the situation?'

FEEDBACK FOR GROUPS

If you have had a team in the simulator it will be more important for them to watch the video together so that they can see how they worked as a team. How they related to each ot her under stress is important.

It will be essential that every member has the same opportunity to reflect and comment in the discussion. No one person should dominate, neither should anyone remain silent.

The focus of the discussion remains the learning outcome that was set before they went into the simulator.

As this team will be experienced and already know each other, they need to focus some discussion on the application and implementation of what they have learned in their normal working environment, so that there is observable improvement in the work place.

CONFIDENTIALITY

The agreement between the faculty and trainees is based on trust. What happens in the simulator stays in the simulator. The faculty want the scenarios to remain confidential so that other trainees can have the learning experience, in the same way that the trainees do not want their performance discussed out of the debrief room.

Points for debate

- How far do you go to make this a 'real-life' situation? Can it ever feel real when the student knows to expect a crisis? Can you actually suspend disbelief? Probably not, but there are great benefits in practising in an environment where mistakes are not a matter of life and death.
- What happens if the 'patient' dies during a scenario? Is this a real-life situation or not? Do patients die during emergencies? Some think the patient should never be allowed to die.
- Should simulators be used for assessment of performance? If a student fails a simulation session, will s/he necessarily be a bad clinician?
- Can, indeed *should*, simulators ever be used for revalidation?
- How far should simulation be used as an educational or training tool? To what extent should trainers depend on it? To what extent is it a necessity?
- Do the benefits outweigh the costs?
- What can and can't we learn by comparing medical simulators with training for airline pilots? Medicine has learned from airline pilot simulations the importance of simulators for non-technical skills. Anaesthetists, for example, started with only technical skills and have now developed to non-technical skill training. What airline industry simulators cannot do is deal with patients. An airliner is not a

living person. With patients there is an unlimited number of things that can go wrong. The cost issue is greater for hospitals.

Summary

Be cautious.

- A simulator is a good tool but it can never replace the patient completely.
- Simulators can be used for the wrong purposes. They should not be used for research because they are anatomically not human. Results from a simulator are not transferable. They can only be evaluated as results from a simulator.
- Good web sites for further information are: www.bmsc.co.uk and www.ssih.org. Also, take a look at the Society in Europe for Simulation Applied to Medicine (SESAM).

Notes for Trainers

Simulators

This chapter lends itself to debate. We suggest that you direct a couple of people to research and review articles for a discussion of any of the issues we have raised.

If you have trainees who are unfamiliar with the technology, you might be able to find a demonstration video of training in a simulator.

Equally, you can ask small groups to decide how they would spend a specific sum of money given to their department for training purposes. It will be interesting to see if different priorities emerge.

CHAPTER 10

Teaching a skill

Introduction

Teaching a manual or psychomotor skill has much in common with other types of teaching, in addition to some unique elements. Planning a skill session is as important as planning any other area of teaching.

Our aim is to produce clinical practitioners who can work at a consistently high level. In order to become proficient each individual must go through the stages of novice, competent practitioner, and ultimately experienced clinician. In order to go from the stage of novice to competent practitioner the student needs to acquire the foundation stones of competence: knowledge, skills, and attitudes (Figure 10.1).

Skills can be divided into two types: technical or manual, and non-technical (an area that covers behaviours, leadership, and team working).

In this chapter we will look at teaching manual skills at novice level and discuss the move from novice to competent. We will also look at what makes you skilled and how this expertise can be acquired.

TEACHING MANUAL SKILLS TO A NOVICE

At the basic level teaching a manual skill is in the psychomotor domain of learning, where we copy or mimic the actions of the expert. We need to demonstrate not only how to perform the skill we are teaching, but why and when to do it. This is why we begin here by outlining an approach to preparation.

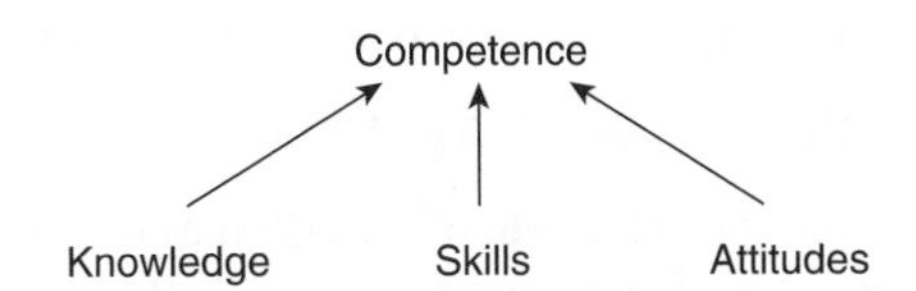

Figure 10.1 The foundation stones of competence.

Planning to teach a skill

Few things produce more anxiety in a student than being asked to perform a clinical skill. They recognize that their partial knowledge combined with lack of experience and dexterity will show them up as inadequate, both to the teacher and to other students. It is almost unnecessary to describe this here—we have all experienced it ourselves. We must consider how we turn this ordeal for the student into a pleasant and positive learning experience.

DEFINING THE AIMS

First, you must recognize that the teacher's and student's aims are not the same, because they have different definitions of success. Take for example the insertion of a tracheal tube. The *student* wants to 'get it in'. If immediately successful 100% happiness follows, and the appropriate box can be ticked. If the student fails to achieve this, misery and humiliation may result.

The *teacher* wants the student to:

- identify those patients in whom intubation may be difficult
- learn to position the head and neck correctly
- maintain a safe airway at all times
- recognize when the tube is in the wrong place, and remove it
- be aware of what else may be happening to the patient or in the room
- recognize when senior help is needed
- be able to keep the patient safe using simple airway support until help arrives
- and also (if possible) to 'get the tube in'!

So before beginning, the teacher needs to explain the aim of the teaching, just as at the beginning of any other sort of teaching.

Look back at the list above of what the teacher wants as opposed to what the student wants.

We know that on the student's criteria of success, about 50% of medical students will fail to 'get it in'. If we use the teacher's criteria of success, most students will be able to succeed with most of the aims. We will also have taught them that the aim of the teaching is airway safety, not technical proficiency, and that the risk to patients is anoxia, not 'anintubia'.

What does the student take away from a good practical session?

- A new understanding of the reasons for performing the procedure, when to do it, and when not to do it.
- The things they have learned by doing the procedure themselves.
- Confidence from having succeeded under supervision.
- Ideas about how they can continue to improve their technique.

IDENTIFY THE LEVEL OF SKILL REQUIRED

Often, the student will never be required to be as good as the teacher. The teacher is probably a specialist, but a trainee nurse or medical student may never need to achieve specialist-level skills. Ultimately, it is of little importance if the trainee psychiatrist is not very good at inserting an intravenous cannula, and the urologist probably does not need to be able to insert a chest drain as well as the trauma surgeon. Trauma surgeons will during their training have many opportunities to insert chest drains. A generalist trainee, however, on a 2-day trauma course, may only have one or two opportunities to acquire this clinical skill. For such a person it is then vital that the skill be well taught, in a simple and memorable way as possible, and that they achieve early success because there may be no more training opportunities.

PLAN THE STRUCTURE OF YOUR TEACHING SESSION

Many teaching opportunities occur because a student arrives unexpectedly. There is no time for the teacher to prepare; this means that if there are special skills you teach regularly you should have prepared your teaching plan in advance.

The plan may include:

- finding our what the student knows, or whether they have attempted the procedure before
- having a clear aim, and telling the student what it is at the beginning
- breaking the procedure down (deconstructing it) into a simple sequence of steps, using the four-stage process outlined below
- evaluating the student's performance, and giving feedback
- summarizing the key learning points
- giving advice about how the student can improve further
- preparing the equipment and any visual aids or hand-outs that will help the student remember—you can easily have a few hand-outs in your desk or briefcase, or in electronic form on a memory stick.
- Asking the students to write down what they found most difficult, what they learned, and what changes they will make when performing the skill in future.

Always focus on steps that are really important, ones that the student is likely to find most difficult, and helping students avoid the most common errors of technique.

Example of preparation for teaching a skill

Skill—taking the blood pressure manually
Students—medical students and student nurses
Knowledge level assumed:

- significance of blood pressure, systolic and diastolic
- position of brachial and radial arteries (may need revision)

Teaching aims:

- choice of correct sized cuff
- correct application of cuff

- measurement of systolic pressure by radial artery palpation
- correct use of stethoscope
- recognition and interpretation of Korotkoff sounds

Common difficulties to focus on:

- using the correct size of cuff
- deciding at what point the diastolic pressure lies

Resources:

- volunteer
- sphygmomanometer
- stethoscope

Deconstruction of technique:

- patient sitting in comfortable position
- estimate length of arm (shoulder to elbow); choose cuff at least two-thirds of this length
- apply cuff to arm without leaving slack
- inflate and deflate cuff while palpating radial artery; estimate systolic pressure
- inflate cuff above systolic pressure
- use stethoscope to listen at the correct position
- listen for and record the levels at which Korotkoff sounds (a) appear and (b) become muffled

Possible visual aid:

- diagram of Korotkoff sounds during cuff deflation

For further work:

- get each student to measure the blood pressure of three other students; construct a table comparing how well the results agree when each student's blood pressure is measured by different individuals
- compare blood pressures in the same students when lying, sitting, and standing.

Starting your skills teaching session

Traditional methods of teaching skills usually involved the old principle of 'see one, do one, teach one', at first on fellow students and then on patients. Here, students are shown a technique by a senior person, then on the next occasion they are left alone to perform the skill themselves, and finally, often after a very few opportunities to do the skill, they were expected to teach other novices! This method was ripe with opportunities to get it wrong, perpetuate mistakes, and hand them on to the next generation! However, it was marginally better than the alternative of 'trial and error' in which individuals were encouraged either to read up the technique in a book or 'have a go'. Neither of these methods is consistent with patient safety, and neither acknowledges that skills require active learning. You cannot just expect people to pick up skills as they go along.

Understanding the skill

Before you start teaching the skill you will need to teach your students some of the theory behind it. It is important to plan this carefully. The content of this first part of the session needs to be focused and relevant, for example if you are teaching how to inject local anaesthetic and steroid into a shoulder joint, you need to give a short introduction to indications, contraindications, equipment, and precautions. Do not give a detailed lecture on conditions of the shoulder, nor on the pharmacology of local anaesthetics or steroids.

Remember that this component can be revised interactively through question and answer if the theory but not the practice has already been covered.

Teaching the motor component

Teaching a skill is a good exercise for the teacher as well as the student! It is often the case that teachers have passed from the competent to the expert many years ago and are able to perform the common manual skills with a minimum of conscious thought. It is often hard to remember what it was like when you could not do the skill! Analysing the steps will enable you to teach the skill more rapidly and successfully. Do you remember your first driving lesson, when you realized you could not change gear and the car lurched to a standstill? You had consciously to follow specific steps for a smooth gear change, steps you never think about consciously now.

Try jotting down all the steps in a simple skill you may do every day, for example inserting an intravenous cannula. Compare your list with these 20 steps.

1. Explain to patient
2. Good light
3. Wash hands
4. Gloves
5. Apply venous tourniquet
6. Skin preparation
7. Comfortable position
8. Identify puncture site in relation to cannula size
9. Open packet in sterile way
10. Fix skin and vein with left hand
11. Inject local anaesthetic if appropriate (for cannula >20 g)
12. Hold cannula firmly and correctly
13. Puncture skin
14. Advance needle 3–5 mm into vein
15. Fix needle and advance cannula all the way in
16. Release tourniquet
17. Occlude vein at cannula distil end to prevent blood spill
18. Remove cap from needle assembly and apply to end of cannula
19. Apply dressing/fixation
20. Flush cannula with saline

Getting resources ready

Having worked out the steps, make sure that you have all the equipment on hand. If you are doing one-to-one teaching on the job, this will not be a problem. If you are teaching away from a hospital, you must ensure that everything you need is in place before you start. This is part of your responsibility as the teacher.

Remember to take copies of your slides, as pictures are helpful in setting the context for the skill. You may also have video clips of the skill to show. If you have written out your script for each stage, take that with you too.

The four-stage approach to teaching a skill

A common and useful way of building up a 'hands-on' skill is the four-stage approach—at each stage the student increases their participation until they can both describe and perform all the component steps. In Stage 1 (Table 10.1) it is important to demonstrate to the student the real-time performance of the skill, but not too fast or visual memory will not be engaged. After you finish Stage 1, check that everyone could see by asking them. There is no point demonstrating a skill if half the group cannot see what you are doing.

The four stages are then repeated with the new learner taking on the role of the teacher. Every student must take a turn at Stage 4. You need to allow adequate time for this. You need to help make the difficult bit easy; if you realize by the third student that they are all making the same mistake, intervene and explain again in a different way.

This four-stage method can only be followed in a teaching room. In some circumstances it may be possible or desirable to vary the method, for example when teaching a student to catheterize the bladder of a real patient. You must be confident of the student's ability to follow instructions. After an oral introduction you may proceed to the learner performing the skill while the teacher gives directions and commentary.

Table 10.1 The four-stage approach to teaching a skill

Stages	Rationale
1 Silent run through by teacher in real time	Learners gain a visual impression of the skill
2 Repeat demonstration with a commentary	Narrative clarifies details
3 Repeat demonstration and learner describes the steps	Builds up memory of the procedure
4 Learner performs the skill	Teacher checks performance and gives feedback

THE NEED TO TEACH INTERACTIVELY

When you are teaching a skill it is important for you, the teacher, to continue to throw out questions to everyone who is observing, in order to keep them involved. Once the students start to go through the four-stage routine, the process can become tedious for those observing, so you use questions to reinforce what you want them to remember: *'Why is she doing that now? What might make you stop what you are doing?'*

As you do this, you are helping the whole group to focus on more than just the skill: get them to consider the context or possible difficulties that can occur. Have your questions ready which begin: *what if …?*

It is particularly important that after the initial stage students are encouraged to ask their own questions: why you do (or do not) perform in a particular way?

THE NEED TO REFLECT

Clearly this is not a one-off process, your students will need to practise many times. Each time that the learner performs the skill it is essential to give useful feedback.

What we see here is learning by seeing, speaking, doing, reflection, and feedback. Students learn best by receiving direct feedback on how they approached and carried out the skill. Use the two questions we keep repeating: What went well? What should you change to improve performance? As the teacher, you need to ask them what they found difficult and whether they feel happy about performing the skill on their own with a patient.

USING MODELS

The four-stage method lends itself very well to learning the basic techniques on model limbs in a skills centre. For a great many procedures models are available, although they vary in how lifelike they are. The idea of learning on models is valuable to the beginner as it allows the learner to examine and familiarize him/herself with the equipment without the stress of a patient waiting or other staff pressurizing for a rapid performance of the skill.

PRACTISING WITH PATIENTS

Patients must be warned about what is going on, then the four-stage method can be used in clinical situations where a number of procedures are performed one after the other. We wrote of ways of how to include patients in your teaching in Chapter 6, page 74.

USING VIDEO RECORDING

If available, a video recording of the real-time performance of manual skills can be a help. It can lead to improvement of communication skills with patients and clearer analysis of technique. We make suggestions in Chapter 12 about how to use a video recording for feedback and it is an integral part of training in simulators, described in Chapter 9. If you, the teacher, do not have time to spend while every student has a go on a model or manikin, a recording, which the students can watch individually or together, can be a reasonable substitute.

Next steps in learning skills

Once the novice has followed the four stages, she or he has acquired a degree of familiarity with the procedure but cannot be deemed to be competent to perform it independently straight away. Once the basics are acquired, it is necessary to repeat the skill many times. This raises a number of questions:

- What is the best way to achieve competence?
- How do we know when a novice has become competent?
- Once competent always competent?

WHAT IS THE BEST WAY TO ACHIEVE COMPETENCE?

For those groups of trainees who need to develop the highest quality specialist skills, it is not enough simply to count the number of times they perform a particular procedure. They need a training programme which focuses on and records all aspects of the skill, including those aspects we have already mentioned: knowledge, manual skills, attitudes, and ultimately the ability to teach the skill to others.

HOW DO WE KNOW WHEN A NOVICE HAS BECOME COMPETENT?

This is an important question to which the answer is of course 'it depends'. Individuals achieve competence at different speeds, depending on their degree of manual dexterity and the rapidity with which they acquire clinical judgment. In order to become good at any manual skill, the trainee needs to perform it a number of times with supervision until they achieve a state where they can be successful 'most' of the time. Even experts do not have a 100% first-time success rate. So our difficulty is in deciding what constitutes 'most of the time'. Once a skill has been 'learnt', it needs to be repeated several times within a relatively short period of time. We also have to be sure that the trainee knows how to manage safely their failure to perform the skill; this may be important for instance in airway skills. Defining success may need some thought, for example is success visualizing the larynx and passing the tube first time? Or is success getting the tube in after three attempts and adjusting the head several times? Both end up with an intubated patient, but the first option may indicate greater skill or experience, or just an easier intubation.

If you are responsible for a training programme, we suggest you read the additional material on learning curves at the end of the Notes for Trainers for this chapter.

ONCE COMPETENT ALWAYS COMPETENT?

Competence, once acquired, does not necessarily remain with the individual. Clinicians may perform skills on a daily basis early in their careers. More senior practitioners may spend less time doing such things. We sometimes describe these skills acquired early in our careers as 'like riding a bike' because generally people who learn to ride a bike as a child can go back and ride after many years without any problem. The truth is that even with riding a bike if one tries to ride after a long interval, progress can be very wobbly at first!

Therefore, if an individual acquires a manual skill during training and that skill is needed again after it has fallen into disuse it may need some refreshing.

Log books: records of training

One way to monitor the acquisition of practical skills by trainees is to keep a record of the number of times they have performed the skill. This is usually referred to as a log book. Exactly what information needs to be collected in a log book may be set down by the training authority. Individual institutions may define the log book data set but basic data should include:

nature and numbers of procedures
assessor's signature
success/ failure
outcomes or complications of the procedure.

You may choose to collect a variety of other information as well.

We deal with examining skills through objective structured clinical examinations (OSCEs) in Chapter 13, Assessing your students' progress, page 170.

> Skills teaching is an integral part of clinical teaching.

Summary

- Get your aims clear.
- Prepare the why, what, how, and what ifs.
- Use the simple four-stage method.
- Reinforce the method with students after initial teaching.
- Keep practising it yourself.

Time to stop and think

- What am I doing well when I teach a skill?
- How can I improve my skills teaching?
- What should I change or add?
- How do I know when I have taught a skill successfully?

Notes for Trainers

Teaching a skill

This is, of course, a practical session but it still needs your trainer input. There is enough material here for two separate sessions. If you only have time for basic training in the four-stage approach, follow points 1–6. In longer courses or for those who are examiners, focus on the other aspects and include the material on OSCEs in Chapter 13, page 160. You need to choose a skill in which your trainees are competent. They are not learning the skill. They are going to learn how to teach a skill and run a skill-teaching session. You need to draw on material from the section on how to prepare, how to teach interactively, and how to manage large groups. Skill centres are often small, overheated spaces, and holding the attention of all students all the time is essential. You need to appear confident and put into practice all the tips on making sure students can see. Then you need to reflect out loud and make all these points explicitly as they all feed into successful teaching of a skill.

Aims

- Understand the principles underlying teaching skills, how individuals move from novice to competent
- Prepare the trainees to run a skill-teaching session using a systematic four-stage method of teaching
- Begin to learn how to plan a skills-teaching programme.

Outline for the basic session

Time: 90 minutes

Resources: equipment, models, suitable room layout, hand-out of sample script, flip chart, plan and equipment for skill stations for Task 2 the workshop, slides for the four stages and the individual steps of the skill.

1 Introduction
2 Trainer input: preparing to teach a skill
3 Task 1: a planning task
4 Trainer input: the motor component and demonstration of the four-stage approach
5 Task 2: workshop on how to teach the four-stage approach
6 Reflection

Additional material

1 Using learning curves as an assessment tool
2 Trainer input: log books: records of training
3 Task 3: devising records of training.

1 Introduction

See Introduction to this chapter, page 121.

2 Trainer input: preparing to teach a skill

See section on Preparing to teach a skill in this chapter, page 123.

3 Task 1: a planning task

15–20 minutes

Choose a skill you regularly perform in your specialty. You are going to train the trainees how to prepare to teach this skill successfully.

The trainees list:

- the essential knowledge they need to establish before they start to teach the skill
- their aims for their future students in a skill-learning session
- the many steps of the actual skill; they must analyse every step including how to pick up and hold the equipment or instruments
- the difficult bits of the skill.

After 10 minutes, encourage trainees to compare their aim and then the steps of the skill.

You put up a slide listing what you think the steps are. Students compare and comment.

4 Trainer input: the motor component and demonstration of the four-stage approach

See section on Teaching the motor component in this chapter, page 131.

5 Task 2: workshop on how to teach the four-stage approach

30–90 minutes

- After observing the four-stage demonstration, trainees are given a different skill and take a few minutes to make notes, which will be their script for a four-stage demonstration of this second skill.
- Trainer listens to a couple of these scripts.
- Explain how the workshop will continue. In small groups trainees will move to the different skill stations. At each one, two trainees will take it in turns to go through the four stages as if they were actually teaching. The rest of the group will role-play being novices.
- When the groups have done this, interrupt and ask those demonstrating what they find difficult and what they forget.
- Ask those observing what they found well done.
- Move the groups around to the next skill station and different trainees take on the role of teacher.

When you or other trainees give feedback, it should only be on how they taught the skill and instructed the novices. There should be no discussion or criticism of the actual technique. This is difficult to adhere to so you, the trainer, must explain this. If you stress that this is a role-play for a teacher with a group of novice students it will be easier. The group comes out of the role to discuss the process.

6 Reflection

After an active session, give your trainees time to write down what they want to take from the session and how they want to teach a skill in the future.

Additional material

1 USING LEARNING CURVES AS AN ASSESSMENT TOOL

- Simple learning curves

Recording success and failure rates gives the trainee a picture of how they are progressing at the skill. This is called a learning curve, which is defined as a curve generated by plotting the success or failure against the number of attempts (Figure 10.2).

In this curve a score of 5 points is given for success and 5 subtracted for failure (completed by the instructor). This is a very simple learning curve from which the success rate, failure rate, and some measure of the rate of learning can be assessed.

Simple learning curves may indicate trainees who are struggling with tasks. Producing learning curves for a large number of trainees will allow some review of the effectiveness of teaching.

In common speech, a 'steep learning curve' means that something was very difficult and many mistakes were made. In the learning curve in Figure 10.2, a steep rise indicates few or no failures—an easy task.

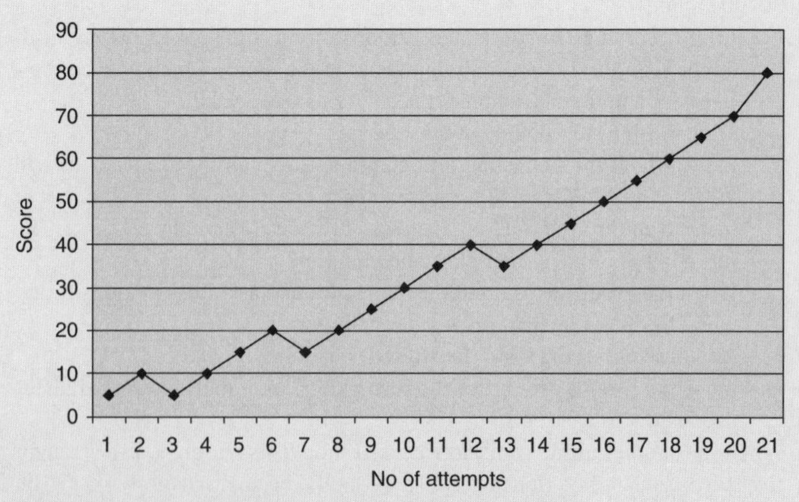

Figure 10.2 A simple learning curve.

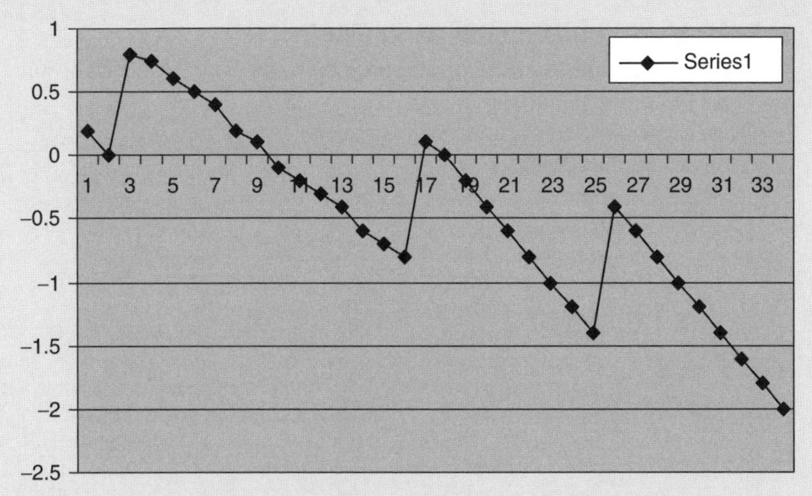

Figure 10.3 A complex learning curve—CUSUM type.

- Complex learning curves

More complex learning curves using an acceptable and unacceptable failure rate can be constructed, but this is a complex process probably more suited to a research project than to use every day in the teaching of trainees. They can be useful in providing assurance of competence to perform tasks solo.

To perform these complex learning curves you can use a statistical tool, CUSUM (the cumulative sum technique). In this technique an acceptable and unacceptable failure rate is defined by discussion with experts. Then a statistical value is given to a success and a failure. An acceptable success rate is defined, and the trainee gets a score for success or failure. Success produces a downward deflection and failure an upward one. As shown in Figure 10.3, failure produces a relatively larger upward deflection than success; the size of the deflections is calculated statistically to reflect the relative importance of failing. Thus in this curve for tracheal intubation, seven successes are required to overcome the effect of one failure.

For more information about CUSUM and learning curves see:

De Oliveira Filho GR. The construction of learning curves for basic skills in anaesthetic procedures; an application for the cumulative sum method. *Anesthesia and Analgesia* 2002; **95**: 411–416.

Schupfer G, Konrad C, et al. Generating a learning curve for pediatric caudal epidural blocks; an empirical evaluation of technical skills in novice and experienced anaesthetists. *Regional Anesthesia and Pain Medicine* 2000; **25**: 385–388.

2 TRAINER INPUT: LOG BOOKS: RECORDS OF TRAINING

See section on Log books: records of training in this chapter, page 129.

3 TASK 3: DEVISING RECORDS OF TRAINING

- Devise a minimum data set for a log book for trainees in your speciality for Year 1 of professional training.
- Now think about the skills needed in the final year of training.
- How would they differ?
- Can they be usefully assessed using a log book?

CHAPTER 11

How to deal with unexpected difficulties—and find solutions

To every problem there is a solution.

There will always be aspects of teaching or a presentation that you can neither fully control nor anticipate. You might find yourself in that situation when you invite questions. We offer a few tips on answering questions and leading a discussion. We follow this with a list of actual problems which we have been asked about by clinical teachers in many different parts of the world. We end with some of their positive comments after they had thought about their problems, found solutions, and returned to their teaching commitment with greater confidence. As with everything, you need to believe there is a solution for every problem and you have the means of doing something yourself. You must be prepared to try out ideas that are new to you, to see if they work.

Taking questions

Always remember that you can take questions at any point during your teaching. If you want to encourage a less formal teaching atmosphere, your students should always feel they can interrupt and ask a question. They may need to because they do not understand something you are explaining. It might be because of medical language.

You should encourage them to ask on the basis that if one needs to ask something, probably others are struggling too.

QUESTIONS AFTER A FORMAL PRESENTATION

If you decide you want to invite questions, for example after a presentation of research or review of articles, here are some things to help you make it work:

- Keep back a summary slide (use the <W> key or <B> key. This means you finish with your take-home message, rather than a distraction from the audience.
- Plan for questions and allow adequate time.
- Always repeat the question for the whole audience to hear.
- If you do not understand what someone is asking, rephrase what you think they mean and check with the questioner.
- Do not say everything there is to say on every question.
- Feel free to ask if anyone else would like to answer the question.
- Keep an eye on the time and on the chairman and tell your audience when you are taking the last question.

If you are not confident about answering questions before a large audience, offer an alternative. Tell people when and where you are available if they have questions.

> You are responsible for the session until it has finished.

WHAT CAN GO WRONG?

- Nobody asks a question: wonderful! Assume you have covered everything satisfactorily and bring everything to a close with your summary. Your audience will be delighted that you have finished a few moments early.
- Everyone puts their hand up: say you will pick three or four. Do exactly that. Choose people from different parts of the room. Then stop.
- There is no time for questions, or just 1 minute left: that is not a problem. Do not take questions.
- Beware the person who stands up and gives a lecture instead of asking a question. This person may know more than you—or thinks they do—and may want to contradict what you have said. Avoid the temptation of a public spat, unless this is something you expected and have thought about in advance. If what is said is in your view clearly wrong, courteously thank the person for their contribution, and say you cannot agree. Ask for a further question from the audience in the hope that it will refocus onto what you do want to say.

Whatever happens, find a positive note on which to end. Show your final summary slide, so that the audience leaves with your take-home message.

Leading a discussion

- What if no one says anything?
  Open your discussion with an open question, then seek opinions from others in the group. It is a rare group that does not have a least one person with an opinion. Do not be afraid of silence, let people think, when you get an answer, don't respond personally but open the discussion up to the group. If they look as if they do not want to participate, be reassuring and encouraging.
- What if one person dominates the discussion?
  You are in charge, so politely thank the person for their contribution and ask another person for their view, preferably in another part of the group or room, so that you shift the communal attention away from the dominating person. It is important that you take action in this situation. There is a negative effect on the rest of the group if one person continually answers. The rest of the group becomes irritated, bored, and loses interest. The whole purpose of active involvement in learning is lost.
- What if the discussion gets away from the point?
  If the discussion is moving too far from the original case or teaching, intervene and politely bring the group back to the point. However much you plan, unexpected things will happen when the group is allowed freedom to speak! Be flexible, be prepared to intervene, to stop and summarize early if necessary, and keep to time. If the discussion is good, suggest that it might continue after the session but don't let it stop you from closing the session properly.

Leading interactive teaching

> You must make every effort to look confident when leading an interactive teaching session and you must show that you are in control.

It cannot be stressed enough that when you appear to be teaching informally and interacting with your students, you must look completely in control of all that is happening. Always be more formal at the start and move to informality, never the reverse. Your approach depends on the age and seniority of the group. If you are too friendly initially, it becomes very hard later if a student has to be told they are not good enough.

SOME GENERAL STRATEGIES

If things go wrong, ask yourself the simple question, '*Was it them or was it me?*'

If you know that you hit a point that was unprepared, or that you were disorganized, then recognize the problems and do something yourself. It may have been some factor outside your control that caused the session to go badly. Do not be down-hearted. Next time will be better.

Whenever you teach in a different way, it is worth explaining at the beginning not only what your aims are, but also how you are going to teach. Tell students you are going to give them time in the middle to discuss in groups; tell them you want them to be thinking and participating; if you ask an open question to the whole group, tell them to raise a hand if they have an answer.

Be very aware of the whole group. Keep looking round and notice who answers, who avoids answering.

Most difficulties are solved by involving the students actively and engaging them through more discussion, group work, and questions. If you can get attention at the start by making your teaching relevant you will keep attention more easily. If they look as if they do not want to participate, be reassuring and encouraging. Tell them what they can do and do not put them down.

It is hard to regain attention if students have been studying in pairs.

Make a noise by tapping the board, clapping your hands, tapping a glass. Wait until everyone is looking in your directions. Start to speak, and if anyone continues to talk, pause and wait for their attention.

- Students start talking while you are teaching.

  Ask them to stop talking.

  Direct a question at whoever is speaking.

  Walk over to that group, and continue teaching from that position.

  Afterwards think how to overcome that problem through changes to your plan, for example stop talking, write up a question, and ask for written answers. You move around the group while they are writing.

  Ask yourself: did I get a good start? Did I start talking before I had everyone's attention?

- The group gets out of hand.

  Most problems arise from sudden loss of confidence, at which point the group takes over. Most new teachers find it hard to be tough and deal with these problems immediately. Perhaps you need to stop and give a written task or a drawing.

- Groups do not work as you expected.

  When you divide students into groups, you have less control over what is happening, and a number of things may go wrong. The major cause of groups not completing the set task is lack of clarity from the teacher about what is expected. Have a pattern whenever you set tasks for pairs or groups:

  You explain what you want them to do.

  Tell them how long they have.

  Show a slide with the instructions which they read.

  After a moment ask if anyone has any questions about what they have to do.

  Leave the instructions on the slide (or written on a flip chart).

  Remember the pause! Start to tell them what you want them to discuss, pause after a couple of words, check everyone is listening, then continue.

  It is surprising how often instructions are given when nobody is listening!

- Students are unclear about how to get into groups!

  Be very directive and divide the students into groups of whatever size you want. You can do this by numbering them off around the room, 1, 2, 3/ 1, 2, 3/ etc. if you want three groups. Tell those who have been given the number 1 to move to a particular place, etc. This mixes up the students.

- Students start moving into groups while you are still talking.
  Only give instructions when you have everyone's attention. It is best to explain the task and then divide them into groups.
- Groups do not listen to each other when they report back.
  Before the small groups begin, explain what sort of feedback you will expect from them, the content and the length, e.g. they will have to give a one-sentence or 1-minute feedback.
  Before the small groups finish, announce to each group how long they have left and now is the time to agree the feedback.
  Get the spokesperson to stand up and speak loudly.
  Take feedback from all groups before you start any discussion. This keeps things moving.
  Use your body! Move to the side of the room or stand at the back, near any who may be talking, and give prominence to the student who is speaking.

Difficulties with student behaviour

- Students absent themselves.
  Keep a list of names and make everyone sign it in front of you when they arrive.
- Students turn up late.
  Firstly, make sure that your own time keeping is good. Start and finish on time. Get into the habit of stopping 5 minutes before the end to allow students time for reflection and/or questions.
  On a long course, at the end of the first session, ask those who were late to let you know if there is any reason why they were late and whether they will be able to arrive on time the following week.
  If lateness persists, explain why you will not tolerate it, it is part of a professional approach to work as a clinician. I have known one trainer lock the door once he has started his training.
- An individual trainee does not like you and shows no interest.
  It is quite possible that a student will not like you. Your aim is not to be liked but to teach well. If you do most of your teaching in a clinical session to just one other person and that person shows no interest in learning, you must persevere and making what you teach relevant.
  Hand responsibility for learning to them. Give them something to look up in advance and get them to tell you the three most important things about what you are doing. If they come unprepared, send them away.
- Students appear bored; they keep looking at their watches.
  One reason this may happen is if you are moving through your material at the wrong pace. If you are going too slowly they will be bored. If you are going to fast they will no longer be listening because you have left them behind. In an interactive session you may be waiting too long for an answer or not long enough. Perhaps what you are teaching is too easy and without an adequate challenge, or is it too difficult and needs clearer explanation?
  Vary the pace and spend more time on difficult sections.

Looking at Pace to Counteract Boredom

Here is a summary on pace, which is an intangible quality of good teaching.

- What is pace?
  clarity throughout the teaching
  clear movement towards goals
  appropriate challenge to all
  interactions
  keeping all students engaged.
- What is it like when pace is lacking?
  the session drags
  students are bored
  students are confused
  the teacher is talking for too long
  no clear goal, no clear structure.
- How are pace and timing linked?
  the lesson moves along
  students are clear as to what they have learned
  you are keeping to time
  you offer a variety of approaches.
- A well-paced session may include the following:
  good resources
  time to think
  adequate challenge through well planned open-ended questions (see Chapter 5, page 54.)
  a variety of ways of attacking a hard topic from different angles and through different teaching methods.

Some Actual Problems

The following are situations that some new teachers faced and had to deal with. They came up with many of the solutions themselves when we met to talk about their teaching experiences.

The time for teaching is too long!

Some people had to teach for 3–4 hours. Nobody can concentrate for that long on one topic taught in one way.

- Plan a timetable in which you include regular breaks.
- Look at the material, and divide it up into sections. Decide which is the most appropriate part for a formal lecture and do this first. Remember the concentration dip, the need to vary the stimulus. You may choose to test this material at the end.
- Plan something interactive for the second hour, with time in groups for discussion.
- Allow students some quiet time to read from a text or journal article. They might prepare some questions for you.
- Include a very visual presentation.
- Finish with some exam question practice.

Put into practice all the suggestions you have read, be creative and you will soon be their favourite and long-remembered, best teacher.

My teaching was just a list of facts.

Sometimes clinical teaching contains a huge amount of factual knowledge that has to be learned. Remember the tip: vary the stimulus. Remember also that the teacher is not the only resource. Try some of the following ideas and think of more.

- Chose the area you think should be already known, start with some general questions and use the techniques described under brainstorming, Chapter 5.
- Choose the most difficult area for the straight lecture. Try to incorporate as many visuals as possible. Give the outline as a hand-out so that the students have to keep filling in the detail as you speak.
- Give a short test on what has been done so far.
- Ask students to read the relevant chapter and prepare questions for each other.
- Give guidance at the beginning and again at the end for what is most important – new learners need to hear this from you. Use your voice to underline what is most important.
- Show up to four slides with facts; click the B/W key and ask what information they have just heard and read.

Everyone was tired including myself.

Most people feel they are tired all the time.

Problem times are early morning teaching sessions and end of day, when you just want to go home. Often the key is preparation so that you, the teacher, feel enthusiastic and ready. Enthusiasm is infectious. A small bribe can be encouraging! Acknowledge tiredness and if necessary ask people to bring a cup of coffee with them, or get them to stand up and move around. Tell them how important the topic is but that you will try to finish promptly if they will kindly give you their full attention.

You know you have prepared a session that will finish 5 minutes earlier than expected and they will be delighted when you finish early. This is part of the relational aspect of teaching, treating each other as equals, meeting expectations, and being reasonable.

Time also passes more quickly if everyone is involved, so include something interactive.

I forgot what to say in my lecture.

A number of new teachers feel they have to learn their presentations by heart. This is a waste of time. Have your outline notes with you.

There is a lack of equipment for teaching a skill.

If the group is too large, divide into smaller groups and give one group a task of background reading, while you demonstrate the skill with what is available to just half the class. Then swap groups.

Try to find suitable video recordings to reinforce what they see.

Always take time to arrange the group so that they all can see what you are doing.

The room is unsuitable and nothing can be moved.

You can move around the room. Find a flip chart because you can move it around.

Most problems are solved by anticipating them in advance!

Those students who raised many of the problems outlined above, returned six months later with the following comments:

I learned to get my timing right.
My teaching aims were met.
My practical teaching improved.
My learners were much happier and more interested.
They asked good questions.
I was clearer.
I had a good structure.
I had good hand-outs.
I worked on being relevant.
I improved my visuals.
I used lots of examples.
Less is more is true!

It takes time to improve your teaching and you will encounter set-backs. But if your aim is to improve then you will.

Time to stop and think

- Do I work hard enough to overcome difficulties, or do I take the easy way out and revert to former ways of teaching?
- How can I prepare to take questions, and gain confidence?
- How can I improve discussion?
- What aspects of dealing with student behaviour do I find difficult? What steps am I going to take to change that?
- How can I apply the section on pace to my teaching?
- If I am honest, what other difficulties do I face?
- How am I going to work out solutions?

Notes for Trainers

How to deal with unexpected difficulties—and find solutions

There is always a solution to every problem.

Some of the difficulties encountered are because some of us have been teaching for many years and find it hard to change. Older teachers on an education course may present some of the problems in such a way as to suggest that your ideas are not possible. It is important that you get such people involved in seeing that solutions are not only possible but essential for improving teaching in the 21st century.

Other difficulties tend to arise from a lack of confidence on the part of new teachers. Even mature adults can become uncooperative if they sense a lack of confidence in a teacher. Managing the behaviour in the teaching room is an important part of teaching. This session tries to talk about techniques to deal with or avoid problems.

With both these groups it is important that you, the trainer, do not come up with all the answers. Try to collect problems and set aside a session in which the trainees work in small groups to come up with their own advice and solutions. The whole philosophy of the course is to give the trainee the tools to be a person who thinks and reflects and tries out different approaches and solves problems. Problem-solving is an important aspect of being a creative teacher.

Our experience is that after initial training, trainees go off inspired and enjoy using new ideas but do encounter problems they had not thought of. Once you have taken these seriously and they have done some further teaching, you will find that they forget about the problems and become much more confident.

A number of difficulties arise from actual students, who are just as indolent or arrogant as they have been in school. Employing a few tricks used by experienced teachers can change attitudes.

You can always choose some of these examples and include them in your initial session. If the trainees learn to anticipate difficulties, they are more likely to realize there are solutions. For example in Chapter 5 How to prepare to interactive teaching, some of the difficulties have been anticipated during the discussion on fears or disadvantages.

Use the material on taking questions according to the make up of the trainees. If they will be presenting at formal meetings and questions are unavoidable, or are an expected part of the presentation, then they must prepare for questions. If, however, the thought of answering unexpected questions terrifies them, they can simply use avoidance tactics, which they have also prepared in advance.

This topic is suitable for small groups or a whole-group discussion when you can collect ideas from the trainees.

Aim

- To get the trainees to solve their own problems and be positive
- To encourage the trainees to take responsibility for their teaching groups and put their solutions into practice.

Outline for the session

Time 40–50 minutes
Resources: hand-out of prepared copies of problems for the groups to read and discuss

1. Positive introduction
2. Small-group discussions
3. Whole-group feedback and comments
4. Reflection on what has been most helpful.

1 Positive introduction

There is always a solution to every problem.

2 Small-group discussions

Take a selection of problems, either from your trainees' own experience or from the chapter, and ensure they provide answers to problems.

Distribute different problems to each group to solve and allow time for a feedback session so that they all hear all the solutions.

3 Whole-group feedback and comments

Ideas spark new ideas and the end result should be positive. After you have listened to a group's solutions, and after inviting others to add suggestions, only now is it time for you to speak from your experience. Offer further ideas, sometimes acting them out, as in the case of moving towards a group that is talking.

4 Reflection on what has been most helpful

At the end, encourage them to make notes on what solutions they want to remember and try out.

Part 4

After you teach: the secrets of on-going success

CHAPER 12

How to evaluate and use feedback to improve your teaching

Good teachers carry on being good learners.

Evaluating your teaching: yourself

WHY DO WE EVALUATE AND ASSESS?

Evaluation and assessment are the tools we use to work out if teaching has been successful and the learner has made progress.

HOW DO WE EVALUATE OUR OWN PROGRESS AND PERFORMANCE?

At different stages in this book we have encouraged you to ask two questions to get you thinking about your teaching:

What went well?

What do I need to do differently to improve?

When you use these questions to evaluate your teaching, and decide what to change, if you implement the changes you will improve. If you get into the habit of reflecting on these questions you will find you continue to improve your teaching.

This method of self-evaluation leading to change in behaviour is based on an experiential model for learning. It is particularly appropriate for adults. It builds on what they already know and on existing experience.

The model we use for adult learning involves a cycle of observing, practising, reflecting, evaluating, and changing, then teaching for real, reflecting, learning some more, changing, practising, reflecting—and so it continues (Figure 12.1). This pattern or cycle of experience enables you to get into the habit of giving *yourself* sensible feedback.

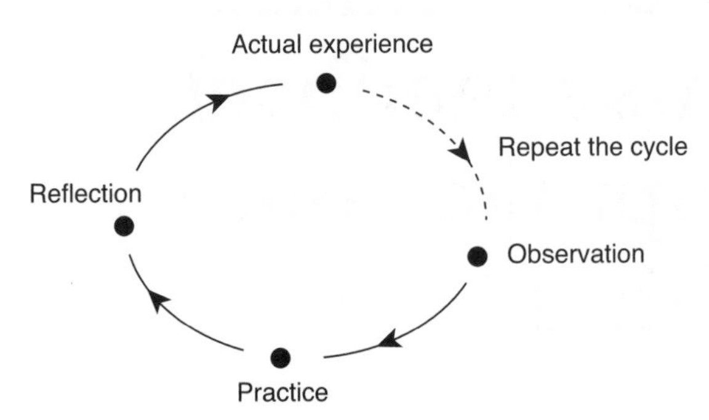

Figure 12.1 A simple learning cycle.

In order to get the most out of learning, you have to experience every part of the cycle. You observe good teaching and receive good information about it; you practise; you receive feedback and reflect, making decisions about what to do differently. You change and that change, we hope, is improvement. This needs more explanation, so we are going to consider learning styles.

Learning styles

WHAT ARE LEARNING STYLES?

Learning styles describe different preferred ways of learning, what we might call our 'learning comfort zone'. Read the next section to see if you have a preferred learning style and fit a 'type' described in the box.

Here is a trivial example to show how we might display our favourite learning style. Imagine you are going to learn to bake a cake. The pragmatist will be motivated by the fact that he or she needs the cake for a birthday party; the theorist will want to watch someone else bake a cake first, carefully following the recipe; the implementer will get going and think about what the ingredients do; the inventors will get the ingredients and mix a cake without a recipe.

Most of us have a style of learning we feel most comfortable with. We limit our ability to learn by sticking to it. Most clinical teaching has traditionally assumed one style of learning. One style of learning is not better than another. In fact to learn as

The four learning styles

Pragmatists

The pragmatists or intuitors enjoy social interaction, they perceive concretely but process reflectively. They like learning by hearing and sharing ideas; they like a challenge, tend not to plan, like immediate application, prefer talking to listening.

Preferred question: *Why?* These learners like reasons.

They need clear goals, and want to know what the point of everything is.

Theorists

The theorists or intellectuals love to deal with facts and ideas; they perceive and analyse more abstractly, they think logically and process reflectively, they need time observing others, and tend to ignore feelings.

Preferred question: *What?* These learners need facts and concepts.

They learn best by having time to consider all the possibilities and do lots of background reading. They need to be encouraged to participate and to take risks.

Activists

The activists or implementers love doing and trying out, working with others. They reflect on experiences and perceive abstractly, but process actively. They want to analyse why things succeed or fail.

Preferred question: *How?* These learners need practical learning experiences.

Reflectors

The reflectors or inventors jump in and try things out, perceiving concretely, processing actively. They are pushy, enthusiastic, driven, like to improvise, to be creative, to make things happen, and to cut through waffle in discussion.

Preferred question: *What if?*

They need to be pushed into becoming more reflective and seeing the importance of underlying principles and concepts. They need to learn to consider alternatives.

clinicians, we need knowledge, practical skills, and positive attitudes, so we must learn in all these ways.

In order for you to be a successful learner we need to take you through a learning cycle in which you participate in all these styles: the theoretical, the practical, and reflection. As teachers, you must apply this cycle to your own teaching (see the steps the trainers follow, Introduction 2 page xvi), and take it into account when you plan students' courses.

You can cover something from each of the different learning styles in a single lecture by using the preferred questions which tend to go with each style; for example explain *why* the topic is important and relevant; give the factual, knowledge-based content (*what*); push the students to apply that knowledge, perhaps through short discussion in pairs (*how*); allow time to reflect on the important things they have learned and encourage them to take that knowledge into the clinical situation.

You need to plan for students to have different experiences over a whole course. You should review the balance of simulating practical skill experience, the simple lecture style or teacher-centred input in which the intellectual learner feels most comfortable, and the real situations with patients; and you must include time to reflect on what has been learned. It is when you integrate all these learning styles that you learn best as an adult.

We have suggested many ways in which you can get your students to be more active learners but they also need to become more reflective and able to evaluate the quality of their work, just as we have encouraged you to do.

On courses to train clinicians and on courses to train teachers, there must be:

- a good mix of theoretical underpinning
- practical tasks
- time to receive feedback and reflect, set targets
- then time to move on round the cycle again (Figure 12.2).

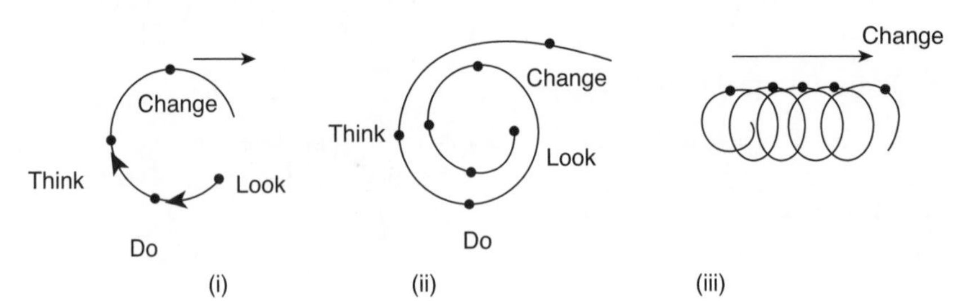

Figure 12.2 A summary of the cycle that leads to change.

When you teach in future, you will continue to evaluate your teaching and continue to develop as teachers because you know how to ask yourself the two simple questions: What went well? What can I do differently or better?

Reflecting in this way is probably not something you do normally! You may spend ages beforehand planning, but very little time after. The secret of lasting success as a teacher is to take time to do this. If you do, you will enjoy the teaching aspects of your job so much more, because you will see you are improving and you will see your students improving. More importantly, they will enjoy your classes because they learn so much.

> Whenever you teach take a moment afterwards to ask yourself: What went well? What will I do differently next time? Why?

Evaluating your teaching: with a friend—paired observation

If you have a friendly colleague, it is a good idea to ask them occasionally to observe you. Give them a specific area on which to focus so that they will know what to do. Give them the two questions: What went well? What should I do differently? Ask them to make notes. When you do this, you will have a good opportunity to reflect with a friend, review how things are going, and gain new insights from a different perspective.

We gave you some ideas about ways in which an observer can help you in Chapter 7.

Evaluating your teaching: using video for feedback

The common uses of video recording are in fields where performance at a clinical skill needs to be evaluated. This is usually in the field of teaching communication skills, interviewing and history-taking techniques with patients, or in developing a skill such as we described in Chapter 10. It is also a useful tool for evaluating your teaching. Using video recordings of your teaching is a good way of developing as a teacher. If you plan to be part of a simulator faculty this is a very good place to begin. You will experience some of the student's feelings in the simulator, and you will have begun to learn how to observe and give feedback.

If you are serious about wanting to work with a colleague who will observe and give feedback then you might think about this extra element—making a video recording and watching it together. If you have done training in a simulator you start with a good understanding of the process.

WHY MAKE A VIDEO RECORDING OF YOUR TEACHING?

- You see what you are doing well.
- You have evidence, for example you can see how long you wait after asking a question.
- You see how students respond and react.

- You become more aware of how you look and sound.
- It emphasizes the fact that you are working with a friendly colleague, not teaching in isolation as you observe video clips together.
- You learn to evaluate your own teaching more accurately.

WHAT ARE THE DIFFICULTIES?

- Embarrassment—you become more aware of how you look and sound.
- Finding the time when you are both free may be difficult: your colleague must be observing while the recording is being made.
- Setting it up and using the equipment may be complicated.

PLANNING

If you decide it would be fun and helpful to go ahead, here are some pointers.

1. Find a colleague who is enthusiastic about teaching. There must be trust between you, and you agree confidentiality.
2. Agree two rounds of observing each other.
3. Agree the detail of the project:
   - (i) dates when you will both be teaching
   - (ii) when, where, and for how long you will meet afterwards to observe and discuss the feedback
   - (iii) how you will be accountable in terms of making changes to your teaching
   - (iv) what would be the best types of teaching to observe, for example a straight lecture, first followed by an interactive session
   - (v) agree the focus, for example the start and finish of a lecture or questioning techniques.
4. Make arrangements for the equipment: the video recorder, a tripod, microphones, and if at all possible a technician who will set everything up and do the recording. Even with much more limited technology—a hand-held camcorder or a mobile phone—it is possible to make short videos on which you can later reflect on the way you teach.
5. Instruct the technician in advance on when you want them to take shots of the students. You can anticipate this from your plan.
6. Formalize the project by telling your colleagues in your department and report back afterwards some of the benefits.
7. You will never show the video clips to anyone else, so decide what you will do with the recordings.

RUNNING THE SESSION

Explain to your students what you are doing. It shows them you take your teaching seriously! They will be pleased to know that you are not keeping the recording of them.

Once you both know the agreed focus for the feedback discussion, the observer makes notes, as outlined on page 151. Keep writing down the time beside your observations as you will then be able to find the place on the recording. Note the time if there is something especially good you want the teacher to see.

DISCUSSING TOGETHER

On completion of the task, the video can be used in different ways. The teacher can watch it alone, and be given time to reflect; then the observer watches to think about what to discuss, or the teacher and observer can go back over the video together analysing particular aspects which the observer has also highlighted in their notes.

The feedback is slightly different from that outlined on page 151. Here the feedback is more positive and should lead to more of a joint discussion about teaching and student responses as you are both watching the video together. There should not be any judgmental elements.

FOLLOW UP

If this works well—and even if it doesn't—do report back to your next departmental meeting. Be specific about the benefits, what you learned, and what you will put into practice. List ways in which students benefited as a result of feedback on your teaching. If others feel they would like to participate, then run a session on observing and giving feedback and deal with all their questions and anxieties. There are notes on this below.

Only ever work with volunteers. You must never impose this on junior colleagues.

Further information is available on the website http://www.curee-paccts.com/mentoring-and-coaching.

How to observe and give feedback

There comes a point where you, as a teacher, should be passing on your teaching skills. The best way of doing this is to give some input to colleagues and then to observe them and give feedback. Every chapter in this book outlines in the Notes for Trainers ways in which you can use the material. It is a good idea to agree to give feedback when those who have done a training session next give a presentation or do some teaching. This section now outlines good ways of doing this.

WHAT IS GOOD FEEDBACK?

It is a conversation between one or more observers and a practitioner about their practice. It is based on an agreement and trust. We want you to be able to learn how to give good feedback in a positive manner in order that the person teaching will gain the tools to evaluate their teaching themselves. When you give positive feedback based on careful observation you promote the cycle of self-directed, independent improvement.

OUTLINE FOR THE PROCESS OF FEEDBACK

The observation and feedback process requires:

1. agreement
2. note-taking and collecting of evidence
3. organization of the evidence
4. a conversation in which the teacher not the observer does most of the talking
5. an agreed way forward.

1 Before observing agree practical details together:
- the focus for the observation; you both need to know which aspect of the teaching is being observed and you will stick to this!
- what the observer will do, for example take notes
- when and where you will discuss afterwards.

2 During the observation the observer:
- sticks to the whole agreement
- is relaxed, smiles, offers encouraging body language
- gathers and writes down evidence for every statement and comment they will make
- is looking at

  the big picture—the impact of the teaching

  the detail and the strategies used

  the responses and learning of students.

Observers must make a note of any or all of the following:
- what is excellent
- the unexpectedly successful
- the main focus of the observation
- things that you think would make a difference
- the lesson aims and whether these are met
- clarity of structure
- quality and use of questions and interactions with the students
- ability to listen to answers
- timing and where time is wasted
- pace and momentum
- reactions of students
- rapport with students
- level of interest and how it is maintained
- clarity of instructions and explanations
- equaly treatment for all students—are they all involved all the time?
- level of expectation, complexity, and challenge
- use of resources: slides, flip chart, board
- preparation and equipment for a demonstration
- management of the students during activities or a demonstration of a skill
- could any section of the teaching have been omitted?
- the opening
- the end of the teaching.

You (if you are the observer) need to plan your notes and write fast! You may design a feedback form. As you collect the evidence, you write down actual words spoken by the teacher/ students.

You are also deciding: what is the most important thing for the teacher to learn about their teaching, to develop or change?

3 Before you have the feedback conversation organize your notes for the feedback! You now have to do some clear thinking to select from the mass of notes some order and priorities which relate only to the agreed focus.
What do you want to emerge in order to help your colleague?
How can you put this into questions so that they can discover this for themselves?
Select, discard, organize, and keep thinking.
Is there anything else that would make a major impact on this person's teaching?

4 The feedback
You enter a formal situation that allows two professional people to discuss a section of teaching as objectively as possible. The focus is on words and actions, not on personality and character.
The aim is that through a discussion of what happened and why, the teacher gains insight into what went on and is therefore in a position to build on strengths and make any necessary modifications to help their students learn better.
Here is a sample set of questions

- Introduction
  Observer—makes a general and positive comment
  Observer—reminds both of the focus of the observation
- The start
  'How do you feel it started?'
  'Did you notice ....?'
  'And why was .... so helpful to XX?'
- The main part of the teaching
  'How did they respond?'
  'Why?'
  'You then moved to ..., did you notice ...'
  'How did X react at that point?'
  'Why did Group Y get on so well?'
  'Did you notice what you said that enabled ....?'
  'What could you have turned into a question?'

Begin to focus your questions more and more on the area you most want the teacher to target and change.
Who is doing most of the talking? This should be the teacher.
Who is doing most of the listening and guiding? This must be the observer.
The observer is basing agreement or disagreement on the written evidence collected.
The observer keeps pressing the teacher to find their own answers and reaches that familiar question: what could you do differently next time?
If you do not agree then you ask another question! Is that the most important thing?

5 Agree the summary
Observer: what do you feel are the most important points to come out of this?
What went well and why? What will you pursue, risk, do more of, develop, modify?

- Why do we always accentuate the positive first?
  we all need encouragement
  we all thrive on praise
  we do not want our colleagues to stop doing the things they do well.

The observer always starts with the positive, however difficult they find that, limits the targets, and seeks to avoid being overly directive.

Evaluating your teaching: information from students

Most formal meetings include evaluation forms on whether the audience approved of the teacher. The resulting data are not targeted and are likely to be depressing. If you are brave, you can give a class you meet regularly your own set of questions so that you receive useful guidance for the future.

When you do this, you are showing the students that you take your teaching seriously and that you want to know what they think. Only do this occasionally. A good time to start is after you do something differently or genuinely need to know their opinion. You might want an opinion on the length of time you expect them to listen, the timing of the coffee break; whether small group discussion is helpful; whether an interactive approach is a good way of revising.

In a subtle way you are beginning to involve future teachers in the evaluative process.

Time to stop and think

- Where do I fit in on the learning cycle?
- Do I really want to improve my teaching?
- What is the best way for me to get feedback on my teaching?
- Should I be taking steps to help others improve their teaching?
- How am I going to do this?

Notes for Trainers

How to evaluate and use feedback to improve your teaching

You need to model good evaluation methods.

There are four areas that you may choose to talk about:

1 Evaluating your own teaching: yourself
2 Evaluating your own teaching: with a friend
3 Evaluating your own teaching: with video
4 Evaluating your own teaching: information from students

If you run a session on evaluation you need a light touch. You should dip into this material and include a little of the theory when it is relevant. One place may be after a couple of active workshops, when you want to reflect on what has been going on and you begin to make explicit the ways in which the trainees are learning.

The learning cycle is something to return to and repeat in more detail, once trainees are comfortable with their training. Some input can only be given as a straight talk, but you should decide how much can be turned into question and answer sessions.

Decide whether slides are necessary Using a board or flip chart to produce the learning circle is more effective.

You must also decide what to omit. Unless you have a long course you will probably omit the section on video and feedback. On the other hand, if you are spending a session with your department looking at ways of improving teaching, you could well focus on that section.

After talking about the concept, a few slides to summarize will be helpful. While you repeat using a different medium, you allow your new ideas to sink in.

The section in this chapter on gaining feedback from students is good for discussion.

Sometimes it is democratic to offer them the various aspects of self-evaluation and ask which one they want to discuss.

Aim

- To give trainees the tools for on-going self-evaluation and improvement.

Outline for the session

Time 10–30 minutes

Resources: slides, flip chart, video clips of unknown teachers—according to material selected

1 Introduction
2 Trainer input.

1 Introduction

Outline different ways of gaining insight into your own teaching.
Get the trainees to tell you the two key questions and write them up.

2 Trainer input

Select from the material. Try to be clear in applying it to the teachers and then getting them to think about how they will apply it to their students.

If there is time, most trainees enjoy fitting themselves into a learning style.

Now decide how much of the following two chapters you want to include.

CHAPTER 13

How to assess your students' progress

INTRODUCTION

When you teach students, what are you trying to achieve? You are hoping to produce competent clinicians who are able to undertake lifelong learning. Competence is dynamic, not something that students achieve and demonstrate on only one occasion, so continuing to learn is a part of professional life. When you teach on one small area of knowledge, keep this bigger picture in front of you. However, there are times during formal training when assessment is necessary. An assessment is useful to student and teacher, as it demonstrates to all that some learning has taken place! This chapter will discuss some of the principles of assessment, and will then look specifically at the use and design of multiple choice questions.

Assessment in medical education

Assessments are used in two ways:

- **Informal assessment**: to check grasp of facts, understanding of concepts, principles, skills, attitudes. This is referred to as **formative** assessment. It informs not only the student of areas of strength and weakness but also the teacher, who can then adjust the content as necessary. Informal, formative assessment can be used to diagnose problem areas and direct the student to areas of their learning that need more work.
  The number of formative assessments to be taken during a course may be set down, and where this is the case they should be spread out over the period of learning.
- **Formal assessment**: to rank students or to make pass or fail decisions This is **summative** assessment. It is based on a formal syllabus. Examinations that come

at the end of the course, summing up what students have learned, are an example of summative assessment.

Both types of assessments are used during training and may be used as an entry level into professional bodies, or for professional self-regulation and accountability. Whatever type of assessment we use, our goals should be to make the assessment accurate, reliable, and timely.

Choosing assessment methods

No single method is comprehensive, so we need to use a mixture of different methods to assess students and trainees.

All assessments must be:

1. reliable—would give reproducible results if used on multiple occasions
2. valid—tests what you want to test
3. cost effective—very important if you are dealing with large numbers of students.

Recently developed types of assessment, such as 360 degree feedback and portfolio-based assessment, are interesting but need to be validated for any group to which they are applied.

When choosing an assessment method or methods think about what you want to achieve.

WRITTEN EXAMINATIONS

These consist of a variety of methods in themselves. They are intended to test factual knowledge primarily. Essays, long or short, have given way to more structured method of written examination such as short answer questions (SAQs). The essay is a less reliable method of assessment because individual variation makes marking difficult. SAQs and short note answers are easier to structure for reliability and validity. They are effective tests of factual recall.

THE EXTENDED MATCHING QUESTION (EMQ)

The extended matching question (EMQ) is a method that extends the MCQ format into a form that is useful for looking at clinical knowledge. Here, a short clinical scenario is described and the student has to match this scenario to a series of potential actions including investigations and treatments. EMQs have become widespread in medical schools.

OBJECTIVE STRUCTURED CLINICAL EXAMINATIONS (OSCEs)

OSCEs have been used in undergraduate and postgraduate medical education for the last decade. An OSCE is an examination intended to test skills, rather than knowledge. It consists of a number of stations, each of a fixed length of time, where a candidate performs a skill and is marked by an examiner. In order to be reliable a large number of stations, between 12 and 16, should be included. This makes it a very labour intensive form of examination, but it has the advantage of greater objectivity and reliability than traditional clinical exams.

Each station needs to be designed for consistent performance. The skill is deconstructed into its component parts and marks are allocated for each part. Setting a pass mark can be difficult, and individual station pass marks may differ. In some models a global pass/fail decision is made by an examiner, in others a set number of marks must be achieved. There should be no 'killer stations' where failure of the station means failure of the examination.

There is a growing literature on the design and use of OSCEs which can guide setters of this type of test.

> Formative and summative assessment tell you whether students have learned anything, and if so what. They also give you feedback on your ability as a teacher. There is a place for both.

Writing and using multiple choice questions (MCQs)

MCQs have become the mainstay of testing of acquired knowledge in education. They are easy to administer and to mark, and can also be analysed statistically to check reliability of the questions. They are relatively cheap and require minimal input from examiners at the time of testing. However, writing good MCQs and maintaining and analysing the bank of questions is a considerable task for any group of examiners. They are time-consuming, difficult to write well, and need regular revision.

MCQs are able to test knowledge at various levels of complexity: simple recall of knowledge with basic MCQs, reasoning and some application of knowledge with more complex, clinically based MCQs.

As with all methods of assessment there are disadvantages.

- MCQs are very poor at testing complex subjects, such as ethics.
- MCQs may in fact test recognition of the correct answer rather than understanding of why it is correct! Students who practise a great many MCQs start to use a technique called 'clueing' which helps them recognize patterns of correct answers without truly knowing and understanding the answer! So they may not even test knowledge.

Many clues are linguistic, based on an understanding of grammar. In English the verbs *is* and *are* give a clue as to the number of correct answers, for example here is a list of answers:

a. USA
b. United Kingdom
c. Australia
d. Romania
e. Argentina

If the question asks: 'Which countries are members of the European Union?', you know immediately that you must tick more than one correct answer. If there is a statement: 'Tick any country that is a member of the European Union', you have to know what is correct.

If the wording of the stem is subtle and complex, the MCQs should not be translated and used in another language as mistakes often occur when this is done.

ANATOMY OF AN MCQ

Before you start to write, you must remember two important facts about MCQs. Firstly, the MCQs should reflect the learning objectives of your course. This is to ensure relevance, validity, and that you are testing what you want to know. Secondly, assessment drives learning. When students find out that there is a question on some small-print aspect of your subject, news will get out and they will all go away and learn up this area, so be sure that your questions cover thoroughly the mainstream of the subject before you introduce more outlying material. Never put in questions on subjects that have not been taught! If questions refer to directed further reading given during the course, it is important to tell students that this material may be included in the test.

THE ITEM

This is the whole question. An MCQ paper is made up of a number of items, usually between 80 and 100 depending on the range of the subject and the time available.

The item is made up of two parts:

1 the stem, a statement or question
2 the options, of which there should be a minimum of four but commonly five.

WRITING THE STEM

The stem is usually composed first and should be a complete statement or question. It must contain the complete information needed to choose the correct option.

- The best stems are short and succinct; for example use
  'The following drugs are metabolized in the liver' not
  'Some of the following drugs will undergo hepatic metabolism as their main route of detoxification and excretion, mark the drugs that undergo this process as correct'.
- If you are designing more sophisticated MCQs to test application of knowledge the stem may be longer.
- The stem must not be misleading or contain a 'trick'.
- Always structure your question for a positive correct answer; for example use
  'The following statements are true' not
  'which of the following statements is not true'.
- Terms such as *always* and *never* should not be used, because in medicine *always* and *never* are very rarely the case!
- Avoid *seldom*, *rarely*, and *occasionally*. They can be difficult to interpret. Use clear statements such as '15% of patients with condition A will also have condition B'.

WRITING OPTIONS

- The option should be grammatically correct and, when read together with the stem, should make a coherent sentence.
- Try not to use eponyms or abbreviations. If you use them, explain them in full.
- If your options are numerical values, order them logically.
- You must vary the position of the correct option. Setters tend to use positions two and three in a five-option question if they are not made aware of the need to vary the position.

If a single correct answer system is used then one correct option, called the key response, and four incorrect options must be composed. The single correct answer MCQ is gaining in popularity in educational circles. Whatever the number of correct answers, the challenge in writing options is to produce plausible but incorrect options. These incorrect options are called distractors.

The distractor:

- can be a correct statement but it does not answer the question set in the stem
- can be a statement that is incorrect but might seem correct to the student
- should not contain 'none of the above' or 'all of the above'
- should be relevant to the stem.

If you use distractors that are very obviously wrong or unrelated to the stem, the question will be too easy.

USES OF MCQS

- To test simple recall, for example:

The following drugs are metabolized in the liver

a. Paracetamol
b. Esmolol
c. Diamorphine
d. Suxamethonium
e. Propofol

(This example has multiple correct answers in common with many medical MCQs.)

- To test application, for example:

A 65-year-old man has difficulty rising from the seated position, but is able to flex his leg. Which of the following muscles is affected?

a. Gluteus maximus
b. Gluteus minimus
c. Hamstrings
d. Iliopsoas
e. Obturator internus

- To evaluate information and problem-solve, for example:

Which of the following actions would decrease the radiation dose from chest CT the least?

a. Decreasing mA from 250 to 125

b. Decreasing kVp from 140 to 120
c. Decreasing the pitch from 2 to 1
d. Decreasing scan time from 1 to 0.5

The questions should discriminate between students. Good students should not be distracted and poor students will be unable to discriminate between correct and distractor options.

AFTER THE MCQS ARE WRITTEN

When you have finished writing your questions and before they are used on students get a colleague to proof-read and review them for you. Ask the question-setting group for feedback to improve your question-setting skills.

Analysis will allow you to look at the difficulty of each item. A good question is one that 50–75% of students answer correctly. Ideally, a question should have only a few items answered correctly by over 90% (indicating it is too easy) or by fewer than 30% (indicating it is too difficult). Individual options can also be analysed to adjust the item difficulty.

There is an excellent UK website (Anaesthesia UK) with many sample questions you can access. To get access you need to register online. If you are outside the UK you can do this on the following website: http://www.frca.co.uk/registration.aspx.

The same principles apply if you are writing EMQs.

SUMMARY

MCQs are a useful way of testing knowledge and they can be designed to test knowledge at all levels of complexity. They are difficult to write well, and require some experience. They should reflect the objectives of the teaching that they test. They should form only part of the overall assessment of individuals and courses.

Time to stop and think

- Do I need or want to get involved in examining?
- If so, what steps should I take?
- Do I need to review any MCQs?

Notes for Trainers

How to assess your students' progress

When you practise writing MCQs and when you give examples, you can prevent arguments by using non-medical examples. This also shows up pitfalls of language and you will find it easier to illustrate linguistic clues.

Aims

- To understand what makes a good MCQ
- To learn to write good MCQs

Outline for the session

Time: 1 hour

Resources: Hand-out 3 (Appendix 4, page 200), board or flip chart, screen and projection

1. Introduction
2. Trainer input: how to write MCQs
3. Task
4. Review of sample questions and reflection
5. Additional task

1 Introduction

- Explain of the terminology of examining—deal quickly with formative and summative assessment

2 Trainer input: how to write MCQs

This is one time when it can be helpful to distribute the hand-out at the beginning of your session. Ask the trainees to read it before you go through and fill it out with actual examples. Your trainees need to be free to ask questions and offer alternatives as you work through together.

3 Task: writing MCQs

- Write three multiple choice questions on any area of your practice. Try to make the questions of increasing complexity. Ask another trainee to critique them for you.
- Write the three items onto a slide and transfer to the main computer.

4 Review of sample questions and reflection

The whole group discusses whether the MCQs are viable and work well. Have a discussion about the way they can go about building a question bank. Stress how time-consuming this is and that it is an on-going project as they must have time to review and validate questions.

5 Additional task: prepare a summative test

Only do this if you have plenty of time and the trainees need practice. Choose the section on your syllabus that you want to examine formally.

Group 1

- Prepare a question for a short answer.
- Produce the key points required in the answer.

Group 2

- Prepare the clinical scenario for an extended matching question (EMQ).
- Produce a series of potential actions, including investigations and treatments you might expect from a medical student.

CHAPTER 14

How to evaluate a course, a conference, or an individual meeting

Make evaluation work for you to improve your courses.

We have looked in detail at how to evaluate your teaching so that you know how to keep improving. Clearly, if you are running a meeting or conference you need to receive feedback from participants and evaluate it yourself, so that next time it will be even better. As the organizer, it is your responsibility to sit in throughout every session (or send a representative) to do your own evaluation and to check that the speakers do what they have been asked.

Why evaluate courses?

Evaluation is necessary in order to find out:

- if we achieved our aims
- which areas to improve
- for Continuing Medical Education (CME) points and official recognition
- which speakers to drop next time.

What needs evaluating?

1. The content:
   formal lectures
   seminars and discussion groups
   practical demonstrations.
2. Practical issues in the programme and organization of the course:
   before—publicity, payment methods, directions, information
   during—programme, timing and length of sessions, venue, meals, timings, exhibitions.
3. The participants:
   what they have learned.

How will you do the evaluation?

You must make evaluation sheets and any MCQs available at the start of the course.

1. The content
   Use key questions: What went well? Was the content relevant? What should we do differently?
- Award marks: 1–5
  1 terrible–5 excellent
- Award a category: A, B, C
  A Good—leave as it is
  B Omit—did not add anything to the course
  C Change—in the following ways ...

2. The programme and organization of the course
   Use key questions: What went well? What should we do differently?
- Award marks: 1–5
  1 terrible–5 excellent
- Award a category: A, B, C
  A Good—leave as it is
  B Omit—did not add anything to the course
  C Change—in the following ways ...
- Group brainstorm
  In small groups or as a large group, ask the two feedback questions (what went well and what do I need to change?) and collect answers on every aspect of the course from quality of teaching to finishing times until they stop coming up with ideas.
  Write down exactly what each person says on a flip chart. Repeat back if necessary for accuracy.
  Do not challenge anything anyone says.
  Use a different colour for different types of points, i.e. things to change, or omit, or improve.

3. The participants
- MCQs
- Observation by trainers during workshops
- Final assignments

How will you get the evaluation forms back?

Allocate time at the end of the course for people to fill in the forms before leaving. You might choose to give out certificates of attendance only in return for the completed form. If you have a responsible group, email the form after the course.

Learn from sensible suggestions; be prepared to make changes.

Time to stop and think

- Do I take adequate note of evaluation of all the presentations? Should I?
- Do I make every effort to get all the evaluation forms back?

Notes for Trainers

How to evaluate a course, a conference, or an individual meeting

This is a short aspect of evaluation which you can do interactively, demonstrating what you mean as you go along.

Aim

- To get your trainees to discover ways of getting helpful evaluation and feedback on courses.

Outline for the session

Time: 20 minutes
Resources; flip chart and pens

1 Questions and answers
2 Demonstration of group evaluation
3 Questions from trainees and further discussion
4 Reflection: questions for trainees

Sample hand-out in Appendix 4 Hand-out 4 page 203
Additional material: how to run and organize a course.

1 Questions and answers

Begin by asking the group why they should do evaluation on a course and what they need to evaluate.

Write up headings as you go.

Distribute the hand-out so they can see if they missed anything.

2 Demonstration of group evaluation

Demonstrate one way receiving group feedback by getting the trainees to give you actual feedback on the course you are running. First, ask them what went well. Their answers should come in any order. Write up all the comments word for word. Then pause and point out the different areas their answer covered.

Ask the second question: what would they change if you run the course again. Receive answers in the same way.

An alternative way of doing this is to divide your trainees into small groups. Give each group paper and a felt pen. As you ask each question, allow them to write down their answers together. You may choose to take in the lists or ask for feedback, to see if the opinions are different in different groups.

3 Questions from trainees and further discussion

Discuss the merits of different methods of evaluating.

It is important that students have the opportunity to ask you questions.

4 Reflection: questions for trainees

Here are some questions you may want to give students to help them to reflect on what and how they have learned on your course.

- What stood out in my mind so far? Why?
- Who is responsible for what is learned?
- What have I done if I have not understood something?
- What am I doing to help me remember important points?
- What is my natural learning style?
- What new ways of learning am I discovering?
- What are the overall learning goals for the course?
- Are the learning aims clearly defined so that I will know if they are fulfilled?
- How are the trainers checking that we are learning anything?
- How will I assess if the course goals have been met?

Additional material: how to run and organize a course

Now is the time to talk to your newly trained trainees about the logistics of them running their own courses. Continue to run the session interactively so that they are doing the thinking as they will have to do detailed planning in future by themselves.

THE FIRST STAGE OF PLANNING A COURSE

Select a small team of two to five colleagues who will share the planning and organization of the course. Start your planning by thinking about:

- who the course is for
- what your aims are for the participants
- the criteria for successful completion, e.g. written work, a presentation, presence in all sessions, participation in groups, leading a small group.

Set a realistic budget and think about sponsorship and costs.

- Who is it for?
  Try to get a group at the same level or with the same background for example all heads of departments, all who are new to university teaching. Alternatively choose people on the basis of whom they teach, e.g. medical students or residents.
- What are your aims for the participants?
  Decide why such a course is important.
  List the outcomes and improvements that are your criteria for success, and which you want to see in the participants by the end of the course.
  Be realistic, select only what you have time for.
  Make sure everyone will have adequate time to complete your criteria for success.
- How long is realistic and when?
  See Appendix 2, page 187 for sample programmes that run for half a day to three weeks.
  Try to avoid times just before professional examinations, unless it is a revision course and therefore very relevant.
- Who will be part of the main training faculty?
  If your professor is a hopeless speaker, find an alternative role for that person. Or find out when he will be on holiday or lecturing abroad. That is the time to hold your course.
  Make sure the course leaders that you want are all available.

  If you are running a course on improving teaching, your training faculty must demonstrate what they are teaching.

Once you have taken these initial steps, seek the agreement and support of the institution head and as many people as possible. If you need sponsorship, ask one person to be responsible for that.

DETAILED PLANNING

Allocate tasks to individuals in your planning team and do not try to do everything yourself.

- Location and venue
  Is the venue accessible? It can be better to find a location remote from where participants live for a course requiring accommodation. In this way your course members will not disappear home or to the hospital.
  Is there more than one room available to divide into groups?

Is the room flexible?
Can tables be moved?
Can you get the room without paying for it?
Who will provide resources—projectors, audio?
Is the black-out adequate?
Is there a photocopier?

- Cost
  Work out the registration fee. Always make a charge, and offer a discount for early enrolment accompanied by the money. Decide on a minimum number of people who must register before a given date. If you do not achieve that, you may need to consider cancelling.
  Set a cancellation fee and a date after which registration fees will not be refunded.
  After working out the precise costs, add a percentage to the fee for contingency of 5–20%. The contingency can be less if you have sponsorship.
  Remember to include the cost of speakers' travel.
  Will anyone need accommodation?
  Set a budget for photocopying and printing.

- Publicity
  How will you let people know about the course?
  In what journals do you need to place an advertisement and how long before the course?
  Should you write an article about the value of improved teaching when the advertisement appears?
  What information do you need to print on the flyers and application forms.
  Who will design and print the brochures?

- Food and drink
  This aspect of any course ensures its success. Adequate breaks and good food go a long way to making people happy.
  It may be cheaper to use a reliable outside caterer.
  Be very clear on what you can afford.

- Clarity on content and programme
  Plan the programme.
  Start time: do people need to travel or are they resident?
  Finish time: always set this 20–30 minutes later than you expect.
  Consider 20-minute presentations followed by a workshop. Try to make some of these interactive.
  Workshops need planning too. Decide on group or pair work and what will be the outcomes.

If you are running an education course, select your training sessions from this book. Do not over fill the programme. Build towards the climax when each person gives a short, individual presentation in the final session.
Allow 5 minutes for each final presentation and 5 minutes for feedback and discussion.
Coffee breaks take longer than you think, especially as it is a good idea to get out of the teaching room and everyone needs to move.
Once you have precise timings for your sessions, allow some flexibility for the following:
The opening and welcome can be delayed by the late arrival of an important dignitary. It can then be further delayed if that person chooses to speak for too long. Relax. The best thing is to agree that your opening teaching session will actually be 20 minutes, but put it on the programme as 30 minutes. It should not be delayed if participants arrive late. It is only fair to those who arrive on time to start on time.
Movement of participants—always expect it to take 5 minutes for everyone to get coffee and 5 minutes for them to return from coffee. Allow a total of 30 minutes, but make sure they all know exactly what time you are restarting. Allocate a faculty member to start gathering everyone 5 to 7 minutes before the re-start.

- On the day
  Decide who does what.
  You need

1. Someone to put up signs to the venue, to welcome, give out name badges, check registration and collect money, hand out evaluation forms, and keep the final certificates safe.
2. Someone to check the rooms, and equipment, and to welcome and look after the speakers.
3. Someone to be available to check coffee and meals. This person is responsible for rounding people up and moving them out of the coffee room in time for the next session.
4. Leaders of small groups who know in advance what they are doing.
5. A time keeper, who will indicate to speakers when they have 5 then 1 minute left, and who will go around groups informing them of the time.
6. A ruthless chairman for the opening session. Their role is to help the speaker to be as effective as possible; to bring the group to attention at the right time; to ensure that the speaker has all the technical help that they need; and that the speaker can be heard and seen by all. This person sets the tone for the whole course. They also have a responsibility to the audience to make sure that the session runs to time as promised by the organizers. They must not allow any speaker to overrun as this is not only discourteous to the audience, and disruptive to the programme, but overrunning sends out a message to other speakers that they can do the same.

- Afterwards

A course organizer has important work to do when the participants have returned home. Make sure you collect in feedback forms.

1 Call a meeting to discuss the evaluation and feedback from the event and make plans for the future. Highlight what you want to improve. Decide what is sensible to act on and what is not! Keep a copy of this.

2 Write a report for sponsors or your university or college department, including:
introduction
background
list of faculty
course and content
evaluation
recommendations for the future
summary
acknowledgements and thanks.

3 Write to your speakers to thank them.

WHAT MAKES FOR A GOOD COURSE?

Here are some comments from courses we have run.

Trainers' flexibility, sense of humour, high expectations of trainee success, treating trainees as equals.

Programme content that was challenging, flexible, which provoked discussion and ideas, which became more demanding as trainees advanced; which offered time to learn from each other and highlighted common problems.

A programme that offered adequate breaks, time for private thinking, left you feeling relaxed, had a good balance of information, practical skills and discussion.

Part 5

Some final questions for reflection

CHAPTER 15

Thinking about values in teaching

Your personal values and world view will affect your view of the teacher, of the learner, and your view of knowledge.

The teacher

- What sort of a teacher are you?
  On a scale ranging from very permissive to authoritarian, informal to formal.
- What sort of teacher do you want to be?
  Think about the qualities of your past teachers.
- Do you care about the people you teach?
  Do you get through your teaching commitment as quickly as possible?
  Do you see your students as individuals?
- What sort of a relationship do you seek to build?
- How do you take responsibility for students' learning?
- What sort of learning community do you wish to establish?
  For example, do you allow your learners to make mistakes?

Most of us are most interested in ourselves, and the impact we make on others; their perceptions of us. We ask: do my students like me? This is not a good question.

Ironically, we will *make* the right impact on our students if our concern is *not* primarily ourselves but them and how best to fit our teaching to their learning needs.

WHAT ABOUT THE TIMES WE TEACH BADLY?

Everyone will teach badly sometimes, when under pressure or not properly prepared. What do you do about those occasions?

The teaching session that follows should be your best, because you now have the tools to analyse what went wrong, to be creative, and follow the steps to prepare properly next time. Let creativity and success develop from failed sessions.

Teachers use words and we have to choose our words carefully sometimes. We may offend or wish to withdraw a stupid comment. Saying sorry is a good way to restore the relationship with your students.

If you are asked a question to which you do not know the answer, then you and the students can aim to find out together. Admitting you do not know everything is more truthful than pretending. The best teachers go on learning.

HOW OFTEN DO YOU PRAISE YOUR STUDENTS?

We all thrive on praise. If students do something well, then tell them. You can change a confrontational culture by showing you notice when others do something well. You will not lose respect, you will gain it. However, do not give praise where it is not due.

The students

- What sort of people do you want your students to become?
  Should they be able to learn from mistakes?
  Do we allow them to make mistakes?
  How can they become confident in their practice?
  How can they be encouraged to pass on good ways of teaching?
  Have they the tools to carry on learning?
  Will they offer better patient care because of how they learn?

Knowledge

- Is knowledge a goal and end in itself?
- Does knowledge improve people or bring happiness?
- How can knowledge be a means to development?
- How does knowledge differ from wisdom?
- If it is true that relationships are at the heart of good teaching, where does knowledge fit in my hierarchy of what is important in life?

All the learning we do in the medical world is aimed at improving the care we give to patients. If we lose sight of this, we defeat ourselves. Every aim we have in teaching needs to reflect this most important goal. Reflection on questions such as these allows us to ensure that we keep on track. It reminds us of the importance of getting our message across successfully.

Notes for Trainers

Thinking about values

You might ask these questions and allow your trainees to think and answer them alone, in pairs, or in groups. The questions can also form the basis for an informal 10–20 minute 'chat' with the group. You may simply give your views on what sort of person you hope to be as a teacher and what sort of clinicians you want to see emerge from your teaching.

This is your opportunity to give an inspiring finish to your course and to refocus eyes on the wider goal for improved teaching, namely improved patient care.

Appendices

Appendix 1: language issues in teaching and training

- A Advice for native English speakers
- B Teaching in a foreign language
- C Working with a translator
- What you need to pack when you teach abroad—a teacher's toolkit

Appendix 2: sample course programmes

- Sample education course programmes
  1. A single lecture
  2. A half-day course improving the presentations of ST3–7s
  3. A one-day programme
  4. A two-day workshop
  5. The first week of a three-week education course
- Sample non-education course programme

Appendix 3: curriculum review

Appendix 4: sample hand-outs

- Hand-out 1 Planning and preparation
- Hand-out 2 Developing interactive teaching skills
- Hand-out 3 Developing MCQs
- Hand-out 4 Evaluating a course or education meeting

APPENDIX 1

Language issues in teaching and training

Always ensure that your audience can hear you easily and speak very clearly.

A Advice for native english speakers

TEACHING NON-NATIVE ENGLISH SPEAKERS IN AN ENGLISH SPEAKING COUNTRY

The rules are simple wherever you teach such a group. This is an ever-increasing issue in the UK with so many overseas students coming to learn or practise medicine.

1. Speak more slowly and clearly than usual. Irish and Scottish accents can be very difficult, especially if delivered at top speed.
2. Use simple language. This means avoid idioms and unnecessarily over-complicated words, for example use give not administer; write down not document; start or begin not commence; count not enumerate.
3. Ensure all new specialist terminology is provided in written form.
4. The language on your slides should be the language in your talk.

Here are some discrepancies within different brands of English.

You hear: white here	the Australian says: wait here
You hear: beer	the New Zealander says: bare
You hear: chicken counter	the Auckland airport announcer says: check in counter
You hear: a hate problem	the Scot says: a height problem

TEACHING GROUPS OVERSEAS WHO USE ENGLISH PROFESSIONALLY BUT NOT OTHERWISE

1. Slow down. Do not gabble. Speak more clearly than you normally do. Rather than asking 'Am I speaking too fast?' when your students may not want to appear to be critical of you nor admit to lack of understanding, ask for a show of hands: 'Who would like me to speak more slowly?' And then try to do so.
2. Keep your language simple.
3. Use short sentences
4. Stick to the words on your slides. Incorporate the words on your slides into what you say.
5. Write up key words.
6. Repeat your questions word for word in small-group teaching. Silence does not necessarily mean lack of medical knowledge.
7. Avoid jokes and idioms.
8. Continue to encourage feedback from your audience. Ask students to query any word they do not understand, e.g. a group in central Europe all heard 'communist' every time we said 'commonest'.

B Teaching in a foreign language

This section is for those who have to present in English when it is not their first language and for native English speakers teaching in a foreign language.

PLANNING

1. Do the preparation in the foreign language.
2. Stick to simple language.
3. Check slides carefully for linguistic errors, if possible with a native speaker. Use the same words on the slides as in your talk.
4. Check carefully how long you take—you may go through with less explanation than in your mother tongue.
5. Do not attempt to tell jokes—let a simple visual cartoon do the humour for you!
6. Practise your opening sentence.

WHEN YOU GIVE YOUR TALK

1. Write out your opening sentence in full and have it in front of you.
2. Ask people to put up their hand if they find a word difficult to make out.
3. Remember to look around and not just at your notes.
4. Try to vary your voice. Listening to a foreigner speaking can be difficult for listeners—vary the speed, stress important points.
5. Stick to what you prepared. Keep to the point.
6. Ask a friend in the audience to be prepared to help if you cannot think of a word.
7. When you teach interactively, ask a native speaker to write on the flip chart.
8. If you speak better than you understand, don't take questions. Thank people for listening at the end and ask them to discuss any points of interest with you afterwards.

9. If you are setting a task then write out the instructions on a slide and/or a hand-out. Ask a local native speaker to read through step by step and ask if everyone is clear about what they do next.

C Working with a translator

> Detailed preparation is the key to successful teaching with sequential translation.

1. The translator should always translate into their own native tongue. Try to find a medically qualified translator who is familiar with medical terminology, and concepts. A clinician with less-than-perfect English is more likely to understand you than a technically perfect translator who does not understand the subject.
2. Experience suggests that you not only need a medical translator who understands your language easily but one who can also translate back into English for you.
3. If at all possible, meet the translator in advance to give them an outline of your talk, a list key words, and time to get used to your voice.

PLANNING AND TIMING

You must plan your presentation to be only half the time allowed on the programme because it will all be repeated in the other language.

SLIDES

If your slides are translated into Chinese, Russian, or indeed any unfamiliar language, you must number them and keep a printout of the numbered slides in English. If you do not do this, you will not know if the audience is seeing what you think they are!

You can have the text in English in a smaller font at the bottom of the slide for you to check that you are speaking to the correct words.

ADVANCE PLANNING IS ESSENTIAL!

If your slides are to be translated:

1. Prepare simple slides and send them in advance for translation.
2. Number and code the slides. Make a printed copy for yourself.
3. Ask the translator to include the number and code on each slide.
4. Request two printed paper copies of your translated slides.
5. When you arrive, staple each translated copy to your original.
6. Stick to what you have prepared.

If your slides are to be shown in English:

1. Prepare simple slides.
2. Give the translator a copy so that he can follow if he cannot see the screen.
3. Stick to what you have prepared.

WHEN YOU GIVE YOUR TALK

1. Remember, it will take twice as long to deliver.
2. If there is only one microphone, give it to the translator.
3. Attempt a few words of greeting in your hosts' language. Do not omit the introductory, courtesy remarks.
4. Ask your audience to query any word they do not understand. This is essential. Your audience will switch off if your translator mistranslates a crucial word. If possible have someone bilingual in the audience to check.

AFTER YOUR TALK

Insist that the translator translates questions for you.

If a discussion breaks out in the audience, insist that everything is translated.

USING A FLIP CHART OR BOARD

1. Prepare your main points and key words.
2. Give one copy to your translator.
3. Give a further copy to another native speaker, who will act as scribe.

Summary of advice on language issues

1. Keep it simple
2. Use short sentences
3. Pause regularly for the translation
4. Enunciate clearly
5. Stick to your script
6. Avoid jokes and idioms at all costs; they do not translate.

What you need to pack when you teach abroad—a teacher's toolkit

Always plan what you need to take for teaching:

- all your electrical equipment and connecting leads
- back up for your teaching material, memory stick, paper printouts of all possible slide shows
- white board writers, chalk, flip chart writers
- Blutac
- pack of biros and pencils
- a simple cloth bag.

This last item is essential if you want to avoid advertising the fact that you are carrying the latest laptop.

Expect a loss of electricity—expect to change from slides to flip charts or board.

APPENDIX 2

Sample course programmes

Sample education course programmes

I A SINGLE LECTURE

Formal:

Always make any lecture on an educational interactive at some point.
Use creative ways of gaining and maintaining the attention of your audience.
Select one topic and include as many examples as possible.
Never spend the entire time showing text slides.

Informal:

Select from the chapters in this book and include a task from the Notes for Trainers, for example
Preparation and planning, setting the tasks on writing aims, Chapters 2 and 3
Top tips for improving presentations with small group exercise, Chapter 7
Aspects of teaching interactively, Chapter 5.

2 A HALF-DAY COURSE ON IMPROVING THE PRESENTATIONS OF SPECIALIST TRAINING 3–7S

08.30–09.00	Presentation: Six steps for good planning Ask after your introduction which of the six steps they tend to ignore; develop that area of preparation; select from Chapter 2
09.00–10.00	Improving presentation and communication skills: as per *Notes for Trainers,* Chapter 7 Coffee break
10.20–11.00	Aspects of teaching a skill—an interactive seminar on how to prepare and think through the steps; how this type of teaching differs from traditional teaching, Chapter 10
11.00–12.00	Either—Improving slides: preparation and presentation; select from Chapters 6 and 8 Or—Using visuals in clinical teaching, Chapter 6

3 A ONE-DAY PROGRAMME

A one-day education course for clinical instructors, e.g. Advanced Life Support (ALS)
Numbers: maximum 10–12 to give each participant a chance to practise teaching under supervision

09.00	20 min	Registration
09.20	10 min	Welcome and aims for the day
09.30	20 min	Why is good teaching important?
09.50	60 min	Tips for effective teaching with a workshop
10.50	20 min	Break
11.10	20 min	Preparing a talk—six steps for good planning
11.30	90 min	Interactive teaching, theory, preparation, and practice
13.00		Lunch
14.00	60 min	Improving your slides, talk and activity
15.00	20 min	Presentation of new slides
15.20		Break
15.35	15 min	Teaching a skill/ how to run a skill station
15.50	60 min	Practical experience at skill stations
16.50	15 min	Summary and certificates

4 A TWO-DAY WORKSHOP

Day 1

Start 8.30

- Why is good teaching important?
- Six steps for planning and preparation
  Workshop 1: writing aims, outlines, and summaries
- Top tips for improving delivery
  Workshop 2: putting the tips into practice
- Making your presentation interactive
  Workshop 3: teaching interactively

Lunch

- Seminar: thinking about curriculum (see slide outline in Appendix 3, page 193)
- Good visual aids—using Power point
  Workshop 4: improving your Power point presentations

Finish 17.00

Day 2

Start 9.00

- Assessment methods: a general approach to assessment and the place of MCQs
  Workshop 5: producing good MCQs
- Teaching and assessing skills
  Workshop 6: putting skill teaching into practice—observation and feedback
- Evaluating your own teaching: a model for adult learning

Early lunch

- Participants all give a 5-minute individual presentation to incorporate what they have learned and receive feedback; this can be done in two separate rooms
- Summary and certificates

NB. Details for workshops are all to be found in the appropriate *Notes for Trainers*.
A session can start with trainer input before a coffee break and continue with the workshop after it.
Finish 15.30

5 THE FIRST WEEK OF A THREE-WEEK EDUCATION COURSE

The value of a three-week residential course is that it allows participants to make progress and think about their teaching in the intervening months.

It is good to aim for about 20 to 24 participants with representatives from a number of different countries.

Not all sessions listed are the same duration—some of the extended seminars take half a day. Education and clinical topics are mingled to vary the stimulus. Interactive teaching is used extensively.

This is an idea of the first of three one-week courses held over a 12 to 18-month period.

Schedule	Notes on content
Day 1	
Aims for course	Not everyone understands why they are here!
Importance of good teaching	Our overall aim is to produce a new generation of effective teachers
Trainee presentations	Trainees start on the first day to get the experience of talking to a group
General interest topic	Example of teaching on a non-clinical subject
Top teaching tips	Outline of basic teaching skills followed by practical workshop
Poster presentation	Trainees present material they have prepared
Day 2	
Education content	
Writing and planning aims	Extended session with teaching interspersed with a variety of tasks
Workshops	Small groups discuss aims and structures for talks
Optional English language class for conferences and international gatherings	
Day 3	
Education content	
Teaching a skill	Extended session with didactic, practical, and feedback sections
Free afternoon	Class needs a break after 2½ long days in a second language

Day 4	
Education content	
Interactive teaching Stage 1	Showing how to do the sort of interactive teaching we have been modelling
Visual aids	An afternoon workshop with practise in preparing visuals and improving slide design ending with presentation of slides
General interest topic: how to introduce change	Preparation for introducing new ideas to their departments
Day 5	
Reflections on the week	Using material in Chapter 15 on values in teaching
Tasks for trainees before Course 2	Homework is required—trainees must now use
(4–6 months later)	what they have learned
Early finish needed! Most participants have to return to another country.	

In the second week, you can build on the topics of basic preparation and using questions, with the material in Chapter 3 on refinements in planning and the second part of asking questions in Chapter 5. This is the time to look at some of the theory and ways of evaluating which you can find in Chapters 12–14.

By the third week, trainees are ready to think about the place of simulators, Chapter 9. They are also ready to learn about observing and giving feedback. At this stage you are introducing different models of small group work, such as we outline in the following example of a course, where students rotate through a series of short workshops.

Sample non-education course programme

A one-day course on a clinical topic: anaesthesia in developing countries
Course numbers: 30 participants

09.30	Registration (coffee available)
	Late start because participants travelling from out of town
10.00	Introduction
	Set the scene, explain how the day will work, lecture: overview of the subject
	Coffee
11–12.30	1 Groups (30 min rotations)
	Participants divided into 3 rotating groups for 3 × 30 min practical sessions
12.45–14.00	Lunch: allow time to move to lunch location, and have a decent break from listening

14.00	2 Seminar groups Paediatrics, obstetrics, and trauma in the developing world Three interactive seminars to combat post-lunch sleepiness Teachers rather than participants rotate to cut down on changeover time
15.10	3 Group scenarios Groups work through a variety of real scenarios/ case presentations Tea
16.20	4 Group talks: experiences overseas Four speakers run seminars about their overseas work: participants must choose any two of these, which they signed up for at the time of arrival
16.50	The Kampala Course Publicity for the one-week course, given by one of our former participants
17.10	Conclusion Summary of the day and take-home message

APPENDIX 3

Curriculum review

This is an outline talk from a slide set for discussing the nature of curricula, how we develop a curriculum and how we deal with resistance to change.

What is a curriculum?

- A cycle of learning
- A dynamic, changing entity
- Systematic sequential learning towards agreed goals

What it isn't

- An academic plan for a total experience which will allow learners to change behaviour

A curriculum must be modified and evolve as required

Step 1 Identify what you want to achieve

What sort of clinicians do you want to produce from your programme?

Who has a say in deciding —faculty, professors, regulating body, professional body, patients, trainees?

Step 2 Identify your learners needs

- Entry level of competence
- Prior educational experience
- Individual goals and priorities
- Attitudes to discipline
- Their assumptions and expectations of the programme

Step 3 Goals and objectives

- More detail on what you want the trainees to achieve
- Set in terms of Knowledge, Skills, and Attitudes
- All the issues in a lesson plan, e.g. less is more, vary stimulus, etc., apply here too

Curriculum objectives should be:

relevant
understandable
measurable
achievable
lead to behaviour change

Step 4 Select the educational methods you will use to deliver the goals

- Lectures
- Seminars
- Practicals
- Tutorials

Think about your resources!

Step 5 Assessment methods

Remember—assessment drives learning

- Have you achieved the goals and objectives you set yourself?
- Plan the exam at the beginning
- Form, e.g. MCQ, written exam, viva, what else?

Step 6 Evaluate and modify the curriculum

May take several attempts to get it right

Circumstances change

Feedback is essential

Evolving dynamic entity

Barriers to change

Fear of loss of control

Who will resist?

Develop strategies to prevent sabotage!

Changing things

Quick and dirty without consultation??

Slow and pleasant?

Change means danger and opportunity

You, the initiators, can influence the perception of others: danger or opportunity?

Changing teaching

Strong support from local leaders helps!

Medical school: Dean, Professors, and others

Summary

Curriculum development is:

- dynamic
- systematic and implemented in a stepwise fashion
- needs built-in feedback systems to lead modifications

All reform will encounter resistance

Try to achieve broad-based consensus from faculty

Provide strong leadership

APPENDIX 4

Sample hand-outs

Hand-out 1 Planning and preparation

Chapter 2 How to prepare efficiently
Chapter 3 How to prepare for a formal lecture

Planning and preparation

Aims

- To help you define the aims of your session
- To define the basic steps necessary for good teaching
- To help you choose the best teaching method

1. Who is this for?
2. Aims: why is this important?
3. Information gathering: what do they need to know?
4. Structure: what order?
5. What do I cut out?
6. How will I finish (and timing)?

Ideas for getting attention

Ideas for maintaining interest

Workshop/ task

The teaching topic: ....

- Consider the group you will teach.
- Write down your aim for that particular group.
- Express your aim in terms of what the students should know or be able to do at the end of your teaching.
- Find a good way of starting.

....

Hand-out 2 Developing interactive teaching skills

Chapter 5 How to prepare to teach interactively

Developing interactive teaching skills

Aims

- For you to develop good question techniques
- For you to become more creative teachers
- For you to develop good interactive teaching skills

Before you teach interactively how do you prepare?

What are good ways of starting an interactive teaching session?

Types of questions

1. Closed questions: usually one correct answer, one word answer, or list, e.g. yes, no

Question words that lead to closed questions are:

What is the purpose of closed questions?

Further examples of closed questions:
What is the incidence of ...?
Give me an example?
Tell me what you do next?
What are the causes of. . . ?
When are you going to . . .?
What is most important in this list?

2 Open questions: there may be no right answer, rather a point of view, an opinion

Question words that start an open question are:

What is the purpose of open questions?

Further open questions:
How would you check . . .?
How do you decide if ...?
What is happening to the patient when. . .?
What evidence do you need before starting . . .?
What assumptions are you making?
Why would you/ not . . . ?

NB. In practice, you will often ask a simple, closed question and then immediately follow up with a supplementary open question.

What are good ways of questioning?

1
2
3
4
5

What are bad ways of questioning?

1
2
3
4
5

What have we learned?

What major change do you want to make to your teaching?

Task 1—Stage 1

- You have been given a topic from the Oxford Handbook.
- With one other person, work out a good opening question.
- Choose a brainstorm method to do this.
- Decide who will lead and who will write up answers.
- You will have 2 minutes to stand in front of the group who will role play a student class.

Task 2—Stage 2

- You have been given a teaching topic from the Oxford Handbook.
- Write out the key points you want your students to learn.
- Turn each statement into a question. You should end up with –five or six open and closed questions.
- Now work with a colleague.
  Ask each other your questions to see if they elicit the answers you expect.
  Discuss the questions and decide on the best ones and why they worked well.

Hand-out 3 Developing MCQs

Chapter 13 How to assess your students' progress

Developing MCQs

Aims

- To understand what makes a good MCQ
- To learn to write good MCQs
  MCQs should reflect the learning objectives of your course.
  Be sure that your questions cover thoroughly the main content of the subject.
  Never put in questions on subjects that have not been taught!

The item

This is the whole question. An MCQ paper is made up of a number of items.
The item is made up of two parts:

the stem, a statement or question
the options, of which there should be a minimum of four but commonly five.

Writing stems

The stem should:

- be composed first
- be a complete statement or question and contain all information needed to choose the correct option
- be short and succinct, unless to test application of knowledge
- not be misleading or contain a 'trick'
- be structured for a positive correct answer, e.g. use 'The following statements are true', never 'Which of the following statements is not true'

Avoid:

- *always* and *never*
- *seldom*, *rarely*, and *occasionally*

Use clear statements such as '15% of patients with condition A will also have condition B'.

Writing options

- When using the single correct answer system one option only is correct, called the key response.
- There must be four incorrect options.

- The option should be grammatically correct with the stem such that when read together they make a coherent sentence.
- Whatever the number of correct answers, you must produce plausible but incorrect options. These incorrect options are called distractors.
- The distractor can be:
  a correct statement but which does not answer the question set in the stem
  a statement that is incorrect but might seem correct to the student
  plausible but incorrect
  relevant to the stem

not very obviously wrong or unrelated to the stem.

- Do not use 'none of the above' or 'all of the above'.
- Avoid eponyms or abbreviations.
- Order options logically if they are numerical values, i.e. smallest to greatest.
- The options must be independent of each other.
- Options must not provide clues as to which is the correct answer.
- Vary the position of the correct option, i.e. use all five positions.

Uses of MCQs

- To test simple recall, e.g.

The following drugs are metabolized in the liver

a. Paracetamol
b. Esmolol
c. Diamorphine
d. Suxamethonium
e. Propofol

- To test application, e.g.

A 65-year-old man has difficulty rising from the seated position, but is able to flex his leg. Which of the following muscles is affected?

a. Gluteus maximus
b. Gluteus minimus
c. Hamstrings
d. Iliopsoas
e. Obturator internus

- To evaluate information and problem-solve, e.g.

Which of the following actions would decrease the radiation dose from chest CT the least?

a. Decreasing mA from 250 to 125
b. Decreasing kVp from 140 to 120
c. Decreasing the pitch from 2 to 1
d. Decreasing scan time from 1 to 0.5

The questions should discriminate between students, that is to say good students should not be distracted and poor students will be unable to discriminate between correct and distracter options.

Task: writing MCQs

- Write three multiple choice questions on any area of your practice. Try to make the questions of increasing complexity. Ask another trainee to critique them for you.
- Write the three items onto a slide and transfer to the main computer.

Hand-Out 4 Evaluating a course or education meeting

Chapter 14 How to evaluate a course, a conference, or an individual meeting

Evaluating a course or education meeting

Aim

- To discover ways of getting helpful evaluation and feedback on courses

Why?

In order to find out:

if we achieved our aims
the areas to improve
for Continuing Medical Education (CME) points and official recognition.

What?

- The content:
  formal lectures
  seminars and discussion groups
  practical demonstrations.
- The structure and organization—practical issues:
  before: publicity, payment methods, directions, information
  during: venue, meals, timings, exhibitions.
- Possible other factors:
  the participants and what they have learned.

How?

You must make evaluation sheets and MCQs available at the start of the course.

- The content
  Use key questions: What went well? Was the content relevant? What should we do differently?
  Award marks: 1–5 1 terrible–5 excellent
  Award a category: A, B, C
  A Good—leave as it is
  B Omit—did not add anything to the course
  C Change—in the following ways ...
- The programme and organization of the course
  Use key questions: What went well? What should we do differently?
  Award marks: 1–5 1 terrible–5 excellent

Award a category: A, B, C
A Good—leave as it is
B Omit—did not add anything to the course
C Change—in the following ways ...
Group brainstorm: in small groups or the whole group
Write down exactly what each person says on a flip chart; repeat back if necessary for accuracy
Do not challenge anything anyone says
Use a different colour for different types of points—to change or omit or improve

- The participants
  MCQ
  observation by trainers during workshops
  final assignments.

Always remember to include the evaluation form at the start of the course.

Index